AN INTRODUCTION TO

CLINICAL

AN INTRODUCTION TO CLINICAL PSYCHIATRY

THIRD EDITION

BRIAN DAVIES

M.D., F.R.C.P., F.R.A.C.P., F.A.N.Z.C.P., F.R.C.PSYCH.

Cato Professor of Psychiatry
University of Melbourne

Section on Child Psychiatry by
WINSTON RICKARDS

M.D., F.R.A.C.P., F.A.N.Z.C.P., F.R.C.PSYCH.

Director, Department of Psychiatry,
Royal Children's Hospital, Melbourne

MELBOURNE UNIVERSITY PRESS

First published 1966
First MUP edition 1971
Reprinted, with amendments, 1973
Revised edition 1977
Third edition, 1981
Printed in Australia at
The Dominion Press, North Blackburn, 3130 for
Melbourne University Press, Carlton, Victoria 3053
U.S.A. and Canada: International Scholarly Book Services, Inc.,
Box 555, Forest Grove, Oregon 97116
Great Britain, Europe, the Middle East, Africa and the Caribbean:
Eurospan Limited, 3 Henrietta Street, London WC2E 8LU

National Library of Australia Cataloguing in Publication data

Davies, Brian Michael, 1928—
        An introduction to clinical psychiatry.
        Index.
        ISBN 0 522 84227 5.
        1. Psychiatry. I. Title.
616.89

CONTENTS

1 Introduction 1

2 The Field of Psychiatry:
Its Development and Present State 3

3 Epidemiological Psychiatry 10

4 Aetiology and Classification 13

5 Psychopathology 19

6 Personality and its Assessment 23

7 History Taking 30

8 Psychiatric Formulation 37

9 Supportive Care 39

10 Neurosis 46

11 Psychotherapy and Behaviour Therapy 57

12 Depressive Illness and its Treatment 66

13 Combined Physical and Psychiatric Illness—Pain—Epilepsy—
The Dying Patient—Grief and Mourning 83

14 Psychosomatic Medicine 92

15 Acute and Chronic Brain Syndromes 98

16 Psychiatric Syndromes in the Elderly 106

17 Alcoholism and Drug Dependence 112

18 Suicide and Attempted Suicide 120

19 Schizophrenia 125

20 Tranquillizing Drugs 133

21 Drug Trials and Placebos 140

22 The Premenstrual Syndrome—Psychiatric
Symptoms and Pregnancy—The Menopause 143

23 Sexual Problems   149

24 Some Aspects of Social Psychiatry   154

25 Some Aspects of Legal Psychiatry   159

26 Consultation–Liaison Psychiatry   161

CHILD PSYCHIATRY BY WINSTON RICKARDS

27 Principles of Child Development   166

28 Childhood Disorders   172

29 Principles of Management   195

Appendixes

1   A Guide to History Taking   207

2   Life Chart   209

3   A Scheme for Memory Testing   210

4   A Guide to Drugs in Psychiatry   213

5   Paperback Psychiatry   217

6   Michigan Alcoholism Screening Test   219

Index   221

ACKNOWLEDGMENTS

I am grateful to my colleagues, Drs Ball, Burrows, Dennerstein, Fielding, Hook, Jones, McLachlan, McDonald,
Meares and Mowbray for their helpful advice. I would
also thank Dr Sidney Bloch for many useful suggestions, and for proof reading. My secretary Sylvia Fraser
is to be thanked for all the typing involved in producing
these notes.

In this edition a new chapter on consultation-
liaison psychiatry has been added, and the chapter on
sexual problems rearranged. Minor alterations have
been made and recently introduced drugs mentioned.

1

INTRODUCTION

These notes are written for medical students with awareness of the limited time available, at present, in the undergraduate curriculum for psychiatry, and with the knowledge that most medical students become family doctors after working for a time in a general hospital.

The management of psychiatric symptoms is one of the family doctor's main tasks, for which he has usually been ill-prepared as a student. The expansion of psychiatric teaching in the undergraduate curriculum, with experience of clinical clerking on patients with psychiatric symptoms, should help to remedy this. The student must learn to think about psychiatry in the same way as medicine and surgery and not to think of it as something abstruse, and quite different from ordinary 'doctoring'. He must learn how to manage the majority of psychiatric problems himself but know when to seek psychiatric advice for his patients. In order to do this he must understand the significance of neurotic symptoms and the supportive care of neurotic patients. He should learn certain basic principles that will guide him in the rapidly developing field of psychopharmacology. The family doctor needs to know something too about psychosomatic medicine, psychiatric illness in the elderly, grief, suicide, alcoholism and sexual problems. Perhaps most important of all he should learn how to recognize and treat depressive symptoms.

Students should be aware that in psychiatry today many differences of opinion exist on such fundamental matters as the aetiology and treatment of many psychiatric illnesses. These differences of opinion reflect a lack of basic knowledge about many aspects of psychiatry. The development in recent years of methods of study which can examine these problems has made psychiatry a rapidly developing research field. In addition, the frequency and social importance of psychiatric symptoms, makes it a growing one for doctors.

These notes have limited aims:

(1) To help the student to take a history in his brief period of clinical clerking in psychiatry and to provide a framework from which he can view his own clinical experience with patients. He must learn a clinical approach rather than any complex system of psychological theories or a detail of psychiatric phenomenology.

(2) To emphasize certain aspects of clinical psychiatry that will be important when he works in a general hospital or in general practice.

The chapters on child psychiatry by Dr Rickards demonstrate principles of the subject, and do not detail specific syndromes. They aim to provide an overview of this important subject.

At the end of some of the chapters a few references are given, to which interested students could refer for further discussion of the subject. For details about individual psychiatric illnesses, reference should be made to one of the following textbooks.

GENERAL REFERENCES

British Medical Journal, *Practical Psychiatry* (London, 1970). Students may find this small book of use when they are qualified.

Freedman, A. M., Kaplan, H. I. and Sadcock, B. J. (eds.), *Modern Synopsis of Comprehensive Textbook of Psychiatry*. Williams & Wilkins (Baltimore, 2nd edn 1976). An American textbook, with chapters by experts covering the whole field of psychiatry.

Gregory, I., *Fundamentals of Psychiatry*, 2nd ed., W. B. Saunders (Philadelphia, 1968). A textbook which combines the British and American approaches.

Hamburg, D. A. (ed.), *Psychiatry as a Behavioural Science*. Prentice-Hall Inc. (Englewood Cliffs, N.J., 1970). A useful paperback overview of present-day psychiatry.

Mayer-Gross, W., Slater, E. and Roth, M., *Clinical Psychiatry*. 3rd ed., Baillière, Tindall & Cassell (London, 1969). The standard British textbook of psychiatry.

2

THE FIELD OF PSYCHIATRY

Its Development and Present State

The word *Psychiatry* comes from Greek words that mean *mind* and *medical treatment*. Psychiatry is an important clinical discipline with strong associations with general medicine and neurology and also with psychology and the social sciences. The word *Psychology* comes from Greek words that mean a *study of the mind*. Psychology is a large field of study, one part of which is medical psychology.

It is not easy to define the field of psychiatry closely. Mayer-Gross, Slater and Roth in their textbook suggest '*that psychiatry is that branch of medicine in which psychological phenomena are important as causes, signs and symptoms or as curative agents*'.

In order to understand the present state of psychiatry it is necessary for students to know something about its past. To start with Greek and Roman psychiatry—the names of Hippocrates, Galen, Aretaeus of Cappadocia, Celsus, Soranus of Ephesus are associated with some of the first recorded clinical observations of psychiatric illness. Hippocrates described one patient with puerperal insanity and another with morbid fears. He described in detail, delirious states and epilepsy and recognized the importance of the brain as the organ of mind.

Psychiatric symptoms were looked upon in the same way as physical illness and a somatic causation for the symptoms was suggested. Greek physicians gave us the first classification of psychiatric illnesses, namely—phrenitis, mania and melancholia. The symptoms of melancholia were described in detail and it was recognized by Aretaeus that the illness would remit spontaneously in time. Treatment of psychiatric symptoms was always physical and Celsus records that attempts were made to bully, torture and frighten patients out of their symptoms. Soranus disapproved of these violent methods of treatment and advised care and comfort for psychiatric patients.

From about A.D. 200 to the 18th century *demonological theories* of mental illness were firmly held; physicians were excluded from the care of mental illness and the insane became the prerogative of the church. The intolerance and persecution which lasted for over a thousand years is difficult to comprehend now. It was, however, almost universally held that the disturbed ideas and thinking of the insane were due to their liaison with powers of evil: they were thought to be possessed by the devil. The punishment was laid down in the Old Testament—'Thou shalt not suffer a witch to live'.

The first recorded execution of a witch in Europe was in A.D. 430. Many thousands were to follow the same fate—500 were burnt within three months in Geneva in 1515. The basis for the persecution of the mentally ill is set out in a treatise by two monks, Kramer and Sprenger titled 'Malleus Maleficarum' (The Witches' Hammer). In this book are described the arguments that lead to the 'proof' of the existence of witchcraft, the methods of identifying witches (including 'stigmata' now recognized as symptoms and signs of psychiatric illness) and finally the methods of torturing and killing them. It is important to recognize that these were not just the views of a fanatic minority, but were widely held. Ambroise Paré, the outstanding doctor of the 16th century, believed that execution was the only 'treatment' for these people. The rare voice was raised against these beliefs and practices. Paracelsus (1491-1541) wrote 'mental diseases have nothing to do with evil spirits or devils—one should not study how to exorcise the devil but rather how to cure the insane—the insane and sick are our brothers'. Johann Weyer (1515-88) made the greatest contribution to psychiatry in the period before the 17th century when he described in detail the various symptoms of mental illness and claimed that mental illness was the proper study of the physician and not the theologian. The widespread acceptance of these views still took time. The laws against witchcraft were not finally repealed in Britain until 1736.

While the witchcraft trials disappeared slowly, the mentally ill during the 17th and 18th centuries were incarcerated in the most terrible conditions 'cared' for by uncouth attendants and punished physically for their 'symptoms'. The places the mentally ill were kept in were essentially prisons, some of which were open to the public as the zoo is now. Mental illness still provoked little interest from physicians with a few notable exceptions. Felix Plater (1536-1614) carefully observed and recorded psychiatric symptoms, yet made no comments about the conditions under which his observations were made. Thomas Willis (1621-75) known for his studies on the blood supply of the brain, thought that punishment was the appropriate treatment for the mentally ill. One striking treatise on nervous disorders was written by George Cheyne (1671-1743) who described his own nervous symptoms in detail.

Eighteenth-century psychiatry was characterized by the many active physical treatments that were used—rotating chairs, shock treatments, blood letting, ducking and starvation—but it was only at the end of this century that the insane were freed from their dungeons. In 1793 Philippe Pinel (1745-1826), Physician Superintendent of the Bicêtre Hospital in Paris, unchained his patients and found that many of their violent symptoms had been due to the manner in which they had been treated. Pinel and his pupil Esquirol (1772-1840) showed real concern for their patients as individuals.

In Britain in the early part of the 19th century, the deaths and disappearances of several patients at York Asylum led to a 'Parliamentary Inquiry into Madhouses' which was made in 1815 and 1816, when a survey was made of all public and private institutions. The appalling conditions prevailing were then brought to prominence. One quotation from the minutes of evidence, illustrates observations made during a visit to Bethlem Hospital (Bedlam):

> In the men's wing in the side room, six patients were chained close to the wall, five handcuffed, and one locked to the wall by the right arm as well as by the right leg: he was very noisy: all were naked, except as to a blanket gown or small rug on the shoulders, and without shoes. Their mode of confinement gave this room the complete appearance of a dog kennel.
>
> In one of the cells of the lower gallery we saw William Norris; he stated himself to be 55 years of age, and that he had been confined about 14 years; that in consequence of attempting to defend himself from what he conceived the improper treatment of his keeper, he was fastened by a long chain. When we saw him, a stout iron ring was rivetted round his neck—while round his body a strong iron bar about two inches wide was rivetted. He had remained thus encaged and chained more than 12 years.

In 1839 John Conolly (1794-1866) introduced the system of *non-restraint* at Hanwell Asylum: 'no form of waistcoat, no hand straps, no leg locks, or any contrivances confining the trunk or limbs or any of the muscles is to be used'.

Gradually conditions improved, patients were treated humanely and were kept occupied during the day. The era of *custodial care* began. Large hospitals for perhaps 2000 patients were built, well away from the cities where the patients lived. There was no active treatment, and these hospitals were usually run by one or two 'asylum doctors' who had little or no contact with the medicine and surgery of the day.

A few men, however, began the real study of psychiatry. In Germany, Griesinger (1817-69) published the first textbook of psychiatry. He held that 'psychological diseases are brain diseases'. In Britain, Henry Maudsley (1835-1918) wrote a number of important psychiatric books. He also believed that psychology was ultimately cerebral physiology. In his will he left money for the London County Council to establish a psychiatric centre for early treatment, teaching and research. The resulting Maudsley Hospital is now the centre for postgraduate training in psychiatry in Britain.

Emil Kraepelin (1855-1926) closely studied the symptoms of patients kept in the asylums and developed a basis of classifying psychiatric illness dependent on phenomenology and outcome. The separation of patients with disorders of mood who improved, from other patients with chronic deteriorating conditions, was now firmly established. There was no active treatment other than waiting for a natural remission, though the value of actively occupying patients was well known.

At the end of the 19th century Charcot (1825-93), the great French neurologist, studied hysteria, believing that hypnosis was a pathological entity characteristic of hysteria. From this clinic Janet (1859-1947) and Freud (1856-1939) began the studies of neurosis that were to produce the most radical changes in psychiatry. Freud's studies led to the development of new theories of the mind and mental mechanisms and provided methods of treatment derived from these theories. These will be described in a later chapter. Jung (1875-1961) and Adler (1870-1937) were also important in this regard.

Bleuler (1857-1939) used Freud's theories to explain some of the irrational thinking seen in patients with severe psychiatric illnesses. He coined the term schizophrenia, describing in his classical monograph all the main features of this mysterious group of illnesses.

Adolf Meyer (1866-1950) had a great influence on American and British psychiatry with his detailed study of the individual patient's development, personality and life. He developed the concepts of 'reaction types' rather than specific illnesses.

The growth and development of psychiatry in the 20th century has been rapid and in particular many effective treatments for psychiatric illnesses were discovered. In 1919 Wagner Jauregg (1857-1940) introduced the malarial treatment of general paralysis of the insane and in 1927 Manfred Sakel (1900-57) introduced insulin shock treatment for schizophrenia. So began methods of effective physical treatments for psychiatric illnesses. In 1933 Meduna (1897-1965) produced convulsions in his patients as a specific treatment and it was soon shown that dramatic results were obtained in patients with severe depressive illness. At first these convulsions were induced by chemicals (camphor, cardiazole) but in 1937 Cerletti and Bini introduced a safe way of producing convulsions electrically.

Thus it became possible to treat severe psychiatric illnesses actively. Illnesses that were known to last for several years if untreated, were dramatically improved within one or two months by convulsive therapy. In 1935 Moniz introduced the operation of prefrontal leucotomy (when the association fibres between the frontal lobe and the thalamus are divided) which, despite its misapplications, has played a significant role in the development of modern psychiatry. These three physical treatments, convulsions, insulin, and leucotomy were all empirical but research began into their possible mode of action.

Between the two wars, the psychiatrist had begun to venture out of the asylum. The large general hospitals developed out-patient clinics and had a 'physician in psychological medicine' who usually took some part in student teaching.

The second world war had profound effects on psychiatry. Experience in the services and among the civilian population showed that neurotic illnesses were widespread. Further, psychiatrists were made to realize that social factors can profoundly influence thoughts and feelings. The actual therapeutic effects of the hospital itself were studied and in 1945 Main described Northfield Hospital as a *'Therapeutic Community'*—where the hospital was not just an organization run by doctors in the interests of their own technical skill, but a community with the immediate aim of full participation of all its members in its daily life. The problem of relationships between patients and members of staff other than the doctors was looked at initially. Experiences of treating groups of patients with psychotherapy at Northfield and Mill Hill began the widespread use of *group therapy*.

In 1952 the first *tranquillizing drug,* chlorpromazine, was introduced and the pharmacological treatment of schizophrenia and other disturbed, restless patients began. Before chlorpromazine and other drugs became available four out of five schizophrenics had to stay in hospital; now few cannot respond to treatment

In 1956 the first *anti-depressive drug*—iproniazid—was introduced and the pharmacological treatment of depressive illness began. In 1958 imipramine was first used in depression and since this time many other drugs capable of modifying depressive symptoms have been synthesized.

These events have led to two major changes in psychiatry:
(1) Active treatment for severe psychiatric illness can now be given by the general practitioner who needs to be fully informed about psychiatry—no longer can these patients be left to the 'asylum doctors'.
(2) The possible way these drugs work has given rise to hypotheses about the nature of schizophrenia and illnesses of mood that can be tested in a scientific manner. From this has arisen a vast expanding research field into the fundamental causes of mental illnesses, which has made psychiatry today one of the most rapidly changing medical disciplines.

Patients with psychiatric illness today usually do not need to be admitted to hospital; treatment can be given either by the family doctor or by the psychiatrist privately, or at the out-patient or community clinic. If hospital admission is necessary then it usually need not be for long. The aim is to treat the patient actively and return him to his family and employment as soon as possible. It is now realized that the large psychiatric hospitals, built in the last century away from the cities, are undesirable. Psychiatric treatment is now *community centred*—private practice, smaller hospitals, out-patient clinics, day hospitals, night hostels, sheltered workshops all are necessary for the needs of the different psychiatric patients. They should all be within the community in which the patients live. Most psychiatric patients can be treated *informally*, i.e. without any certification procedures, yet in many countries legislation still lags behind these advances in psychiatric treatment. With regard to *community care* (one of the important areas of psychiatry today), the field of *primary*

7

medical care is not the same as traditional general practice. Primary medical care uses a team of health professionals, in a defined community, rather than a single family doctor. Such care gives special attention to *prevention* (including health education and screening for early disease) *supportive*, and *rehabilitative* care.

It should now be clear why psychiatry is important to medical students. The family doctor is increasingly concerned both with patients with psychiatric illnesses he treats himself and also with patients who have been treated at psychiatric out-patient clinics or hospitals.

Despite these advances, which have been so recent, the absence of pathology or an agreed psychopathology has led to the development of several schools of psychiatry. These will be mentioned briefly, as fundamental differences of opinion about the causes and treatment of individual patients can be found between psychiatrists working in the same city. Similar basic differences would not be found in medicine or surgery today. The *extreme contrasts* between psychiatrists are found in those whose approach is essentially a *psychodynamic* one and those whose approach is an *organic* one. The former emphasize psychological factors in aetiology and use psychopathological theories that stem from Freud. Treatment is basically psychotherapeutic and physical treatments receive less emphasis, especially in the treatment of neurosis. The latter emphasize genetic and constitutional factors in aetiology and lately biochemical theories of severe psychiatric illness have been to the fore. Treatment is usually either by drugs or by other physical methods. Formal psychotherapy is eschewed.

In an expanding field of study, where psychodynamic theories have been so illuminating, where physical treatments have been so valuable, and social measures so important, it is not easy to steer a middle path between diametrically opposing views. It is only careful investigations that can answer many of the present-day problems in psychiatry that are the centre of differing opinions.

SUMMARY

In this chapter the history of psychiatry has been briefly reviewed. The rapid changes that have occurred in the last 30 years have outpaced legislation, hospital building and medical student training.

REFERENCES

Hunter, R. and Macalpine, I., *Three Hundred Years of Psychiatry*. Oxford University Press, 1963. This book contains extracts of original papers and books. Their presentation with introductory notes by the authors gives a particularly interesting account of psychiatric history.

Thomson, R., *The Pelican History of Psychology* (Harmondsworth, 1968). A sound paperback on this subject.

Ziboorg, G., *A History of Medical Psychology*. Norton & Co. (New York, 1967). The standard book on the history of psychiatry.

3

EPIDEMIOLOGICAL PSYCHIATRY

Epidemiological psychiatry may be defined as that branch of psychiatry which is concerned with the incidence, prevalence and distribution of mental disorders. There are two main types of epidemiological enquiries:

(1) *Prevalence studies* and (2) *Aetiological studies*.

PREVALENCE STUDIES

In recent years, a number of investigations have shown that the problems raised by psychiatric illness will present themselves frequently to doctors in every field of clinical practice.

To start with some general figures: there are half a million patients in psychiatric hospitals in the United States and half of these have chronic schizophrenia—an illness of essentially unknown origin. In most countries half the available hospital beds are, in fact, occupied by such schizophrenic patients. One child in five will, at some time in his life, need expert help because of neurosis or personality problems, while one child in twenty will be hospitalized during his life for severe psychiatric illness. This is most likely to happen over the age of sixty. It has been shown that in groups of sick people something like 30% will be found to be suffering from psychiatric symptoms. It has also been calculated that 80 million working days are lost each year in industry in Britain because of neurosis.

Such generalizations are made on the basis of findings from epidemiological surveys which for any type of illness depend upon:

(1) defining the individual 'case', and

(2) defining the population in which the 'case' is found.

Epidemiological studies in psychiatry are particularly difficult because of the different ways there are of defining a 'case'. There is throughout the world a lack of uniformity in psychiatric classification that depends essentially on the diversity of aetiological theories and the paucity of objective measurements. In a survey of tuberculosis, radiological or bacteriological results would help define a 'case'. In a survey of blood pressure, recording of B.P. under standard conditions can be performed, and if desired some arbitrary standard of 'hypertension' defined. No such tests are available if we set out to measure the incidence of neurosis, depression or schizophrenia in a population.

Most of the figures available are derived from *admissions to psychiatric hospitals*. First admission rates are used to indicate the *incidence* of the particular psychiatric illness while the number of patients in hospital, with that illness gives us a measure of its *prevalence*.

However, when a whole community is studied the limited value of such hospital statistics is realized. A large part of the 'iceberg' of psychiatric illness is never detected using psychiatric hospital records. A number of such studies on whole communities has been done—they show particularly that hospital records are no guide to the incidence of neurosis and personality disorders which are the main problems for the family doctor. They also show that even illnesses like schizophrenia can be present without there having been a recorded hospital admission. The surveys show too the importance of depressive illness and educational subnormality.

In Sterling County, Nova Scotia, Leighton and his colleagues found that using the American Psychiatric Associations Diagnostic Manual's definitions of psychiatric disorders, two-thirds of the entire adult population would, at some time of their lives, have suffered from some type of psychiatric disorder. At the time of the study, at least half of the adults were suffering from such a disorder. They also found that there were as many non-hospitalized cases of severe psychiatric illness, organic brain syndromes and mental deficiency in the community as there were in the hospitals. The great bulk of psychiatric symptoms found were, however, associated with psychosomatic, psychoneurotic and personality disorders.

Surveys of general hospital practice and the work of family doctors also emphasize the importance of psychiatric illness in present-day medical practice. Thirty per cent of patients attending medical out-patient clinics have been shown to have a psychiatric illness only, while another 10-40% of patients have both physical and psychiatric disorders. (Here the problems of depressive illness are particularly important.) Similar figures were obtained in women attending gynaecological out-patient clinics where one conclusion was that 'emotional tensions outweighed physical malfunction and disease as a cause of illness in the patients seen'.

The College of General Practitioners in Britain showed that 30% of the new patients seen by the family doctor have neurotic symptoms. Dr John Fry working in a practice in suburban London has found that he sees 5-10 patients a day with psychiatric symptoms. Middle aged women are most common. Single men and widows are seen twice as frequently as would be expected from their numbers in the community at large. Only 2% of these patients were ever admitted to a psychiatric hospital, though he referred 5-10% to psychiatric out-patient clinics for further advice. Sixty per cent of these psychiatric patients were neurotic patients (usually with anxiety and depressive symptoms); 20% had psychosomatic illnesses; 5% had personality disorders while 3% had severe psychiatric illnesses (12% were classed as 'miscellaneous'). It is important to emphasize that only 3% of the family doctor's patients have schizophrenia, dementia or mental subnormality though the social problems presented by these patients are often considerable.

The student will see from these figures that his main concern in practice will be with neurosis and personality disorders, psychosomatic illnesses and depressive illness.

In general, treatment for psychiatric illnesses, although often empirical, is now effective. On the whole patients with psychiatric illness can be helped to as great an extent as in general medicine, and new treatments often bring dramatic improvements in a short space of time.

AETIOLOGICAL STUDIES

Aetiological clues are sought by examining variations in illness rates within a population and their relationship to environmental factors. Recent work on schizophrenia, for example, has concentrated on defining the interplay of possible genetic and environmental factors. Studies that look at the genetic contribution to schizophrenia have aimed to separate out hereditary effects and a childhood environment altered by the presence of a schizophrenic parent. Children of schizophrenic mothers, brought up in foster homes, have been followed up and compared with controls from the same foster homes but without a schizophrenic parent. The findings that 5 of 47 such children developed schizophrenia compared with none of the controls provide evidence to support the view that there is an important genetic factor in schizophrenia.

Other studies have looked at relationships between childhood bereavement and later depression and attempted suicide; birth order and personality development; Down's syndrome and epidemics of infective hepatitis. Studies on the epidemiological aspects of suicide are described in chapter 18.

SUMMARY

Epidemiological studies in psychiatry look for aetiological clues and give information about the rate and patterns of psychiatric illness in the community.

The difficulty of assessing the prevalence of psychiatric illness in the community is emphasized.

Studies show that at general hospital out-patient clinics and in general practice, psychiatric symptoms are among the most frequent that doctors encounter.

Neuroses, personality disorders, psychosomatic and depressive illnesses are the main problems for the general practitioner.

REFERENCE

Dunham, W. H., 'Psychiatric Epidemiology in Medical Ecology', *International Journal of Psychiatry*, vol. 5 (1968), pp. 124-46. A useful overview of the subject.

4

AETIOLOGY AND CLASSIFICATION

With our present understanding of psychiatric illnesses *there are always multiple causative factors to be considered in each patient.* After a full psychiatric history has been taken these factors can often be graded in some sort of hierarchical order, where one is considered more important than another. However in the present state of our knowledge it is wise to recognize that *many of the most important factors are as yet unknown* (e.g., in schizophrenia, senile dementia, severe mood disorders).

Students should first recognize the difference between *aetiology* and *psychopathology*. Aetiology refers to general causes of illness and such causes are often conveniently considered as intrinsic or endogenous (i.e. due to hereditary and constitutional factors) and extrinsic or exogenous (i.e., due to physical events or mental experiences).

Psychopathology is an area of theoretical psychiatry where psychological symptoms are explained in psychological terms, e.g., an hysterical paralysis can be 'explained' by using such concepts as 'dissociation' and 'conversion'. The development of psychopathological theories, particularly by Janet, Freud, Jung and Adler in the early part of this century, opened up a new dimension in psychiatry. Previously psychiatry had tended to be a catalogue of symptoms and signs. Psychopathological theories gave a new understanding about the meaning of the symptoms and gave possible explanations about why symptoms were present. Psychopathological theories depend upon ideas about mental development and mental processes in which notions (often borrowed from physics) of competing forces (or drives) and 'mechanisms' are used. *Central to the core of most of these theories is the concept that symptoms are due to the person's defences against anxiety.* These theories will be discussed in chapter 5.

There is a popular idea (fostered by novels, films and plays) that psychiatric disturbances often have one emotional cause that the patient has forgotten, but if the doctor can help the patient to remember this then symptoms are at once relieved. This notion has no counterpart in everyday psychiatric practice. It will be mentioned that aetiological considerations always involve a number of factors, while treatment is usually a complex gradual process.

AETIOLOGY
The Intrinsic Causes of Psychiatric Illness

Hereditary predisposition to the major psychiatric illnesses is transmitted genetically and twin studies have shown the importance of hereditary factors in schizophrenia and severe mood disorders. The patient's personality make-up and his body build are both a reflection of genetic endowment.

Some patients who develop schizophrenia have previously shown a schizoid personality, i.e., they showed such traits as shyness and eccentricity. Patients who develop an obsessional illness may previously have shown marked obsessional personality traits (i.e., rigid, obstinate, parsimonious people). Regular mood variations may be part of the personality of patients who develop depressive or manic illness. Some of these patients too have a pyknic body build (rounded thickset configuration).

① stingy

② short, thick, stocky build

It is important to emphasize that most people with these personality features do not in fact develop schizophrenia, obsessional states or illnesses of mood, but if they do become psychiatrically ill they are likely to do so in that way (see chapter 6).

The study of heredity and psychiatric illness has been due largely to Kallmann in the United States and Slater in Great Britain with their studies of the incidence of particular psychiatric illnesses in uniovular and binovular twins.

Affective Disorder

Slater has suggested that manic depressive illness is determined by a single dominant gene of weak and variable penetrance. Thus, half the children of a parent with this illness will inherit the gene. In some, there will be no visible effects; others will have a cyclothymic personality, while approximately 10% will develop an illness like their parent.

Schizophrenia

No single genetic theory fits all the facts. One theory suggests a partially dominant gene, another a recessive mode of inheritance.

Mental Retardation

Severe types of mental retardation are due to a number of different pathological conditions. A few are due to rare recessive genes, e.g. phenylketonuria. Most patients with mental retardation make up the lower end of the curve of distribution of intelligence in the community and are usually born to parents who are not themselves mentally retarded.

Dementing Illnesses

Huntington's Chorea is due to a single dominant gene, as is Pick's disease.

Phases of Development

Certain intrinsic phases of development are important in considering causes of psychiatric illnesses. Puberty, pregnancy, the puerperium and the climacteric are such phases when psychiatric symptoms are not uncommon.

The psychological and physiological changes occurring at these times can all be incriminated in considering why some patients develop symptoms or are worse at these times, while still other patients improve.

The Extrinsic Causes of Psychiatric Illness

These include *physical events* (trauma, toxic and metabolic factors, infections, neoplasms, degenerations)—particularly when these affect the brain; and *mental experiences,* which cannot be easily classified. Students should realize that individuals react selectively and differently to their environment, e.g. they will be aware of the different effects that an impending examination produces in a group of students.

In any particular psychiatric patient students should consider aetiology under the following headings:

(1) the patient's hereditary and constitutional make-up
(2) psychological factors in early life
(3) factors operating at the present time—be they physical, social or psychological.

In everyday psychiatric practice *these three groups of factors all operate together,* but therapeutic intervention may depend particularly on a close knowledge of (3). It should again be emphasized that in psychiatry today many important aetiological factors are still unknown.

In clinical work, it is helpful to ask: 'Why has this particular patient become "ill" in this way, at this time?'

CLASSIFICATION

Knowledge about the causes of many physical illnesses has grown enormously in the last 50 years. In contrast to medicine and surgery where diseases are classified on the basis of their known pathology, the diagnostic classification in psychiatry *depends upon grouping symptoms and outcome* rather than upon a known cerebral pathology or an agreed psychopathology.

There are many ways in which psychiatric illnesses can be classified, but there is no right or wrong way, merely useful and less useful for a particular purpose. Students need only know broad groups of illnesses, and the following system deliberately simplifies many clinical difficulties. It will, however, be a useful frame of reference for clinical work.

Psychiatric illnesses can be grouped into two large groups:
(1) *An Organic group* and (2) *A Functional group.*

ORGANIC DISORDERS

In these illnesses, pathological lesions are regularly associated with the symptoms. These disorders constitute about a quarter of all psychiatric illnesses admitted to hospitals, and are of increasing importance with ageing populations. They are caused by the usual traumatic, toxic, neoplastic, infective, degenerative or metabolic factors, and the clinical syndromes will be described later. There are two characteristic groups of symptoms found in patients with these organic disorders. These are:

Memory disturbances
Changes in consciousness

Both these symptoms will be discussed later. These organic disorders can be subdivided into:

An acute brain syndrome (which is reversible)
A chronic brain syndrome (which is irreversible)

The whole field of *mental deficiency* could also be grouped with this organic group of illnesses, but for convenience it is usually considered separately.

FUNCTIONAL DISORDERS

Most patients with a psychiatric illness have a *'functional'* illness. Here, no organic pathological basis for the symptoms has been established—though it is likely that neurophysiological and biochemical abnormalities will eventually be found to be present in the more severe forms of illness (schizophrenia, severe depression and mania). Patients with these functional illnesses do *not* show the memory disorder or the changes in consciousness characteristic of the organic group. These functional illnesses can be sub-divided in a number of ways. The following is a simple scheme:

Illness of Mood (Affective Disorders)

Depressive illness (a common illness)
Manic illness (an uncommon illness)

Schizophrenia

This term probably includes a number of separate disorders that have certain common clinical features. At present, the essential causes of these illnesses are not known.

Personality Disorder and the Neuroses

(1) Some people have abnormal personalities, but are not 'ill' nor do other people obviously suffer because of them.
(2) Where the patients themselves suffer from the disorder, the group of conditions is known as the *Neuroses*. This group of conditions includes fairly well defined but uncommon syndromes, such as obsessional illness and hysteria. Most commonly, neurotic patients show symptoms of anxiety and depression (see chapter 10).
(3) When *society* suffers from the patient's abnormal personality, the disorder is called the *sociopathic* or *psychopathic* personality.

To complete the classification two other groupings are necessary: *Psychosomatic Illness,* and *Mental Deficiency.*

The words *neurosis* and *psychosis* are often used as if each represented two entirely distinct conditions. The words are used differently by different psychiatrists so that they are best avoided—*particularly as a diagnostic exercise.*

In general, however, *neurotic* patients have symptoms that are mild, but are often chronic. These symptoms, e.g., anxiety, mild depression or phobias are familiar to most people. Neurotic patients are usually not a danger to themselves or others, and can usually be treated without admission to hospital.

Psychotic patients are usually patients with severe symptoms that are foreign to most people, e.g., hallucinations, severe depression or excitement. These patients may be a danger to themselves or others and usually need admission to hospital for treatment of the acute symptoms.

THE NATURAL HISTORY OF PSYCHIATRIC ILLNESSES

The natural history of the different psychiatric illnesses is an important field of study; more is known in this regard about the more severe disorders, i.e. those patients who are admitted to psychiatric hospitals. More detailed information about the patients with psychiatric problems treated by their general practitioners would be particularly valuable.

Illnesses of mood (depression and mania) clear up in varying periods of time (usually several months) but they tend to recur.

Schizophrenic illnesses usually run a chronic course with gradual personality deterioration. Except for the possibility of suicide, life expectancy is not affected.

Acute brain syndromes are reversible and usually do not last for more than a week or so. Chronic brain syndromes show a gradually deteriorating clinical picture until death occurs, in usually not more than a few years.

In general, neurotic symptoms improve over the course of a few months, but they tend to recur throughout the patient's life. The behavioural disturbance associated with hysterical and psychopathic personality disorders occurs in adolescence and early adult life.

Obsessional symptoms are either periodic or very chronic. Hypochondriasis and depersonalization are two groups of symptoms that are difficult to alter.

Psychosomatic illnesses are characterized by attacks of symptoms that can sometimes be related to emotional problems.

SUMMARY

Aetiology in psychiatry always involves the consideration of multiple factors, some of which are still unknown.

Three main groups of factors are involved:

(1) hereditary and constitutional factors
(2) psychological factors in early life
(3) psychological, physical and social factors operating at the time of onset of the illness.

In most patients these three groups of factors operate together.

Problems of classification in psychiatry are discussed. Classification at present depends upon a consideration of symptoms and outcome.

A simple classificatory scheme is given.

The general outcomes of the main psychiatric illnesses are outlined.

5

PSYCHOPATHOLOGY

Psychopathology uses psychological concepts to explain the nature and origins of symptoms and interpersonal problems. The development of psychopathological theories in the last seventy years has been of immense importance to psychiatry, particularly in the understanding and treatment of neurotic symptoms. Students will find it easier to understand the nature of psychopathology if the beginnings of the subject are outlined.

Psychopathological theories began in the second half of the last century with attempts to explain the phenomena of hysteria, using psychological concepts such as 'suggestion'. Charcot (1825–93) the French neurologist, studied hysterical patients with neurological methods and believed hysteria to be a disease entity with definite signs. He held that hypnosis was a pathological phenomenon seen only in hysteria. Janet (1859–1947), a pupil of Charcot, found that the phenomena of hysteria were capable of being explained using *psychological* terms. In order to explain phenomena such as anaesthesia and amnesia seen in these patients, he suggested that there was a *'dissociation in consciousness'*, so that certain memories were cut off from the main stream of consciousness, though they could be demonstrated by hypnosis. Janet's concept of dissociation helped to understand and explain hysteria and hypnosis. The theories were described in psychological terms and were the basis for later psychopathological studies.

While it would be valuable to be able to explain the phenomena of hypnosis and hysteria in physiological terms, to date such explanations have been less helpful to clinicians than psychopathology. Janet's theories did not explain satisfactorily *why* the dissociation had occurred in hysterical patients, and it was Freud (1856–1939) who, in attempting to answer this question, developed fundamental notions of a dynamic psychopathology which have been so valuable in clinical psychiatry.

In 1893 Freud and Breuer, while treating an hysterical patient, showed that her amnesia was explainable as the result of repressed feelings that the patient could not tolerate at a conscious level. Hypnosis was used as a method of bringing these hidden memories into consciousness and of helping the patient by this ①'abreaction'. Soon Freud abandoned hypnosis altogether and developed a method of investigation based on 'free association', coining the term *'psychoanalysis'* to distinguish his method from other abreactive or hypnotic techniques.

Psychoanalysis makes use of dream material and other manifesta-

19

① the reliving of an experience in such a way that previously repressed emotions ass. c̄ it are released.

tions of unconscious processes and relies heavily upon analysis of the transference, that is, the re-experiencing in the analytic situation, of earlier, but now inappropriate emotional states and their consequent projection on the analyst.

To explain his observations Freud grouped mental function into three areas:

(a) a central largely rational, regulating function—the ego

(b) an unconscious group of functions—the id—pressing for expression, and thought of as sexual and aggressive in nature.

(c) a judging moral, punishing and rewarding function (also largely unconscious)—the super ego. This is held to arise from learning in childhood from both parents and from the society the child is brought up in.

Freud also developed the concepts of a ① dynamic unconscious, separated from consciousness by the force of repression, which is met with clinically as resistance.

Freud's work helped to explain the puzzling irrationality of neurotic symptoms and behaviour. The everyday language of psychiatry has borrowed heavily from Freudian terminology. *The understanding of the emotional and non-rational nature of the unconscious and its effects on everyday behaviour was a most important advance. Freud also showed that neurotic symptoms have a meaning in terms of the patient's hopes, wishes and fears.*

Freud continually modified and developed his own views and since his death his theories have been continually modified.

Students who wish to understand this area of study should start by reading Freud's *Introductory Lectures on Psychoanalysis* and *The Life and Work of Sigmund Freud* by Ernest Jones (Penguin Books).

Central to our understanding of neurotic symptoms is the notion of *conflict* and *anxiety*. Emotional forces may run counter to conscious wishes so that a conflict situation arises. Biological needs and drives may be in conflict with the parental and societal ideals, and this expresses itself first as *anxiety*. *Physiological studies show that the body maintains homeostasis in adapting to various changes in the environment. The comparable psychological steady state is maintained by mental mechanisms which protect against anxiety. These mechanisms operate automatically and without conscious recognition. If they fail excessive anxiety ensues and clinically anxiety symptoms are complained of.*

A simplistic account of these mental mechanisms is given through a few everyday clinical situations.

Denial is a commonly used defence mechanism. Without being aware of doing so, the patient excludes from awareness some painful fact or feeling. Bereaved people and patients with acute serious physical illness can show denial. Bereaved patients can later blame the doctors or hospital showing ② *projection* of the bereaved person's own

② Help protect ourselves from recognizing our own "undesirable" qualities by assigning them in exaggerated amounts to other people

To conceal a motive from oneself by giving a strong expression to its opposite — Reaction Formation

① A motive ğ cannot be gratified in one form is directed into a new channel.

hostility to the dead individual, and showing *displacement* of the guilt feelings which are commonly found in bereavement.

Repression is the basic defence mechanism by means of which unwelcome thoughts and feelings are excluded from consciousness. In analytic treatment repression expresses itself in 'resistance'. Analysis of this resistance is an important part of the treatment. The defence mechanism of repression should be distinguished from *suppression*, which unlike the defence mechanisms mentioned is a conscious, voluntary attempt to dismiss unpleasant thoughts, feelings or bodily sensations.

Sometimes patients present a rational explanation to account for behaviour when the real motives are unacceptable, unrecognized and unconscious. The real motivation, being unacceptable remains repressed and the behaviour is explained away or *rationalized*. Unrecognized and unacceptable impulses may be *sublimated* into culturally appropriate forms of expression, e.g. the sportsman may channel otherwise unacceptable aggressive drives into determined play.

One characteristic aspect of sick individuals is *regression* when the patient reverts to modes of thought, feelings or behaviour appropriate to an earlier stage of that person's development in an endeavour to cope with the anxiety arising from being ill. A sick person can revert to a dependent mother/child relationship with a nurse, and may develop magical expectations of the doctor, who is seen as an all-powerful parent.

A clinical example may help students understand these 'mental mechanisms'.

A young woman has developed a paraplegia after a car accident. Following this she does not seem to be particularly unhappy, she *represses* her feelings of loss and despair. She talks about being able to ride her pony in a few weeks, that is, she *denies* the fact that she is crippled for life.

As these early defences dissipate others come into play. She begins to feel a diffuse sense of anger and frustration at her plight but she attacks the medical staff, that is, she *displaces* her anger. She talks also about how unhappy another of the patients is, and she *projects* her own unhappiness on to another.

It is important to once again emphasize that these mental mechanisms occur without conscious control. While 'patient' examples have been used they also occur in doctor and nurse.

It is not possible here to describe further psychopathological theories. It is true to say that at the present time, such theories have outgrown the basic observations and assumptions on which they are based. Different schools of psychopathology have developed and have tended to view their own theories dogmatically. Concepts are talked about as if they were 'real' and not man-made explanatory ideas. It is difficult to use such ideas and theories to establish an hypothesis that can be tested. For this reason scientific studies in this field are lacking.

These psychological mechanisms are only one of the ways that the human organism copes with stressful experiences. In recent years studies of coping, interpersonal problem solving, and adaptive behaviour have been made: for example, how do individuals cope with severe illness in themselves or the death of a loved one? These studies on the ways of human adaptation are important present-day research topics in psychiatry.

REFERENCES

Brenner, C., *An Elementary Textbook of Psychoanalysis*. Doubleday Anchor Paperback (New York, 1974).

Brown, J. A. C., *Freud and the Post-Freudians*. Pelican (Harmondsworth, 1974). This book explains the main principles of Freud's theories and reviews the main development of the theories in America and Britain.

Freud, S. (trans. Riviere, J.), *Introductory Lectures on Psychoanalysis*. 2nd ed., Allen & Unwin (London, 1949). Still the best book to start to read about psychopathology and psychotherapy.

Jones, E., *The Life and Work of Sigmund Freud*. Pelican, 1974. A biography of Freud by his senior British colleague.

Wollheim, R., *Freud*. Fontana/Collins, 1974. A clear brief account of Freud's life and works.

PERSONALITY AND ITS ASSESSMENT

The term *personality* refers to an individual's unique qualities—his enduring features of intellect, behaviour, temperament and mood that have developed as a result of his basic genetic endowment and his growth in a unique environment.

The study of personality, its development and measurement is a large field of psychology. Psychologists consider personality structure as a combination of clusters of traits in the three main areas of ① temperament, character and intelligence. Personality and physical constitution are also correlated and measures have been devised that give an index of body build. In general, personality traits are assessed by psychologists by questionnaires that have been scientifically drawn up. Other objective tests (e.g., of persistence, of conditionability) may also be used. The names of Cattell and Eysenck are associated particularly with these methods of personality analysis. The Rorscharch test—an analysis of the patient's interpretations of a number of standard ink blot patterns—has been used clinically but it is not a reliable test, i.e., different testers tend to come to different conclusions about the significance of a patient's responses. In general, psychologists use personality tests to investigate the nature of personality and its relation to other factors.

The clinician is more concerned with descriptions of personality in the everyday practice of psychiatry. As will be mentioned, one of the main functions of history taking in psychiatry is *to obtain a picture of the patient as a person*. In order to do this the patient (and his relatives) are asked to trace his development from childhood to adult life. The patient is encouraged to talk freely about his attitudes to his father, mother, siblings, wife, children, friends, school, employer, health, money, intellectual activities, hobbies, habits, etc. The way he talks about all these aspects of his life will reveal certain personality features that are useful in the clinical understanding of the patient and his problems.

Many psychiatric patients show features in their personality that can be recognized as important in respect to their present illness. *In these patients the illness seems to be exaggeration of certain marked personality features.* It is important, however, for students to recognize that many people who are not psychiatrically ill show similar features, and the presence of the features that will be described does not imply that the person will necessarily become psychiatrically ill.

The actual details of theories of personality development cannot

23

be entered into here. They are of great interest but are complex and contradictory. In general it is thought that emotional problems in infancy and childhood can result in a failure of normal personality development. Certain personality features will however be described, and students must learn to recognize them in clinical work. *They are not independent and several may be seen in the same patient.*

Trying to answer the question, *Why is this person like this?*, is an interesting exercise that cannot, usually, be solved with any degree of accuracy but some general considerations are given with each personality feature. These considerations will range from psychodynamic factors to conditioning theories.

ANXIETY FEATURES

Anxiety is a universal human experience and both the feeling state and the somatic accompaniments are well known responses to 'stress'. People whose personalities are marked by anxiety are tense, restless people who feel anxious at times when other people would not. Their anxiety 'threshold' is low. These people at interview have moist hands and skin and are unable to relax, they have wide pupils, and complain of palpitations and of the feelings of anxiety or tension that come on with minor stress. They will say that they have been like this since childhood, and as a rule have limited their activities to avoid all situations that they know will produce anxiety.

People like this may say that their mother was always anxious, and observation of an over-anxious mother and her child can readily show how a child could become anxious in everyday circumstances. Anxieties about specific objects—animals, foods, certain situations— can also be learnt in this way from the mother. Other patients give a story of a grossly disturbed childhood, with death or separation of parents, or frequent parental quarrels.

OBSESSIONAL FEATURES

People with marked obsessional features tell their story carefully, weighing each word before speaking. They describe their symptoms, and their previous medical attention in such minute detail that the history becomes a slow laboured story. An obsessional person will be punctual and will be correctly and neatly dressed (often with a mackintosh and umbrella—in case it rains). Obsessional people are orderly, meticulous, clean, precise perfectionists who adhere to time-tables and are dependent on daily rituals. They become anxious if these habits are upset in any way. They are unduly sensitive to interference; they are persistent, thorough but obstinate people. They usually find it difficult to delegate work, and desire perfection not only in themselves but in their families (difficulties often developing with adolescent children). Spending money is often a problem, and some obsessional people are very particular about spending small amounts of

24

money, though they find it less difficult to write a cheque for a larger amount. They are sometimes collectors. Bowel habits are important to these people who become upset if these are altered temporarily.

Some of these obsessional features are part and parcel of Western civilized life, and many of the best workers in certain occupations, e.g., banking, accountancy are helped by possessing these personality features. Sometimes promotion presents difficulties however, as obsessional people as a rule are overconcerned with details. They find it difficult to look at a problem distantly and decision making can be made difficult by the doubts that obsessional people have. They often have trouble sleeping, as they tend to ruminate about the day's events and cannot exclude them from their mind. A satisfactory sexual life is unusual when these features are marked, particularly in women who usually find intercourse distasteful.

Stern, strict parents who emphasized regular habits (particularly bowel habits) are likely to have obsessional children. Psychoanalytical studies in depth of obsessional patients have suggested that obsessionality is a defence, particularly against aggressive feelings. Psychologists point out that these people are introverted and readily form conditioned responses. As has been mentioned these personality features are not uncommon and it does not mean that such people will become ill. However, the following illnesses are often seen in people who show marked obsessional personality features:

Depressive Symptoms

These are an important problem and may follow a bereavement, the development of a physical illness, promotion or more minor problems.

Obsessional Symptoms

The above personality features do *not* interfere with the patient's life, and it is only the development of obsessional symptoms that do this (chapter 10). Their development may be a sign of the presence of a depressive illness.

Anxiety Symptoms

These symptoms—and particularly concern over health—are common; again these may indicate the presence of a depressive illness.

Psychosomatic Illnesses

Peptic ulceration, ulcerative colitis, migraine and asthma are probably more common in people with marked obsessional personality traits.

HYPOCHONDRIACAL FEATURES

People having marked hypochondriacal features in their personality make-up usually have obsessional traits, but it is useful to draw attention separately to the person who is always concerned about his and his family's health. These features can be often traced back to childhood, and parental oversolicitude over childhood illness may be found. Pains are magnified and the patients appear to have a great need for sympathy. Athletes, medical students and the elderly are frequently over-concerned about the significance of minor symptoms.

NEURASTHENIC FEATURES

People with these features become easily fatigued at times of stress. Again they are often associated with obsessional features. Other members of the family may show similar features.

MOOD VARIATIONS

Some people have a characteristic mood level. Some are persistent pessimists who view every event in this light; others are persistent optimists, happy active people whose mood level seems to be fixed above the normal. Both these types of people, and others with a more 'normal' mood level, are liable to regular mood changes that have been present from childhood. These mood changes are usually towards depression and occur at regular or irregular intervals of weeks or months. Less commonly is the mood elevated, and less frequently still do people have cyclical changes of lowering and elevation of mood. If these do occur in some regular sequence the term *cyclothymia* is used. These people are often of thick set (pyknic) body build, and are liable to develop the severe mood disorders of the corresponding type described later. In many of these people constitutional causes for the mood abnormality seem the most likely explanation.

THE HYSTERICAL PERSONALITY

The problems involved in the use of the terms hysteria and hysterical personality will be discussed in chapter 10. It will be emphasized that the words unfortunately tend to be used when the observer meets some hostility-provoking behaviour from a patient.

People with an hysterical personality show a theatrical quality to their general behaviour, particularly in group situations where they seem to have a need to impress others, to gain prestige or sympathy. There is a striking contrast between the way they express their feelings and their actual feeling experiences. The contrast may be shown particularly in the sexual sphere, where their appearance and behaviour may be sexually provocative yet a mature sexual relationship is impossible. Like children, people with these personality features can temporarily live in their fantasy world.

Chodoff and Lyons (1958) have given a composite picture of the hysterical personality: 'the hysterical personality is a term applicable to persons who are vain and egocentric, who display labile and excit-

① able but shallow affectivity, whose dramatic attention seeking and histrionic behaviour may be to the extreme of untruthfulness, who are very conscious of sex, sexually provocative, yet frigid and who are dependently demanding in interpersonal situations.' The authors comment that this is a caricature of femininity as described by men!

It seems likely that the hysterical personality as described above is dependent on constitutional factors and also on personality development in early life.

SCHIZOID FEATURES

③ *Not revealing ones thoughts and feelings readily; Discreet*

It will be mentioned in chapter 19 that about half the patients who develop schizophrenia, have since childhood showed a number of personality traits that are called collectively *schizoid*. *Shyness* and *eccentricity* are perhaps the cardinal features of these traits. These people prefer their own company, are② timid and ③reticent. There is a tendency for them to have an asthenic body build. Constitutional factors are probably the most important ones in producing the schizoid personality.

② *easily alarmed, not bold, shy*

PARANOID FEATURES

People with many paranoid features readily attribute hostile or aggressive motives to others. They are extremely sensitive to interference and this may be associated with ideas about their own importance. Deaf people and migrants (especially those with language problems) are particularly likely to show these features.

SOCIOPATHIC (PSYCHOPATHIC) FEATURES

The word psychopath is used rather differently in different parts of the world. In Britain, it is used to describe people who show persistent anti-social traits. It has been defined as a persistent disorder of personality (whether or not accompanied by subnormality of intelligence) which results in abnormally aggressive or irresponsible conduct. The key to the diagnosis is the *persistent social maladjustment in the absence of the traditional clinical psychiatric entities*. Three main problems are associated with psychopathy (they are usually combined):

(1) delinquency
(2) aberrant sexual behaviour
(3) drug addiction and alcoholism.

Constitutional factors are probably most important in the aetiology of these personality features. Attention has been drawn to the high incidence of maternal deprivation (see chapter 24) in psychopaths. Psychologists point to the fact that these people tend to be extraverted and form conditioned reflexes poorly. As ageing occurs, changes in the sociopath's personality patterns do occur; the clinician (unless he works in prisons) does not meet with these personality features after the age of 40-45. It is unfortunate that like the word 'hysteria' the term psychopath is used to describe patients whose behaviour the individual doctors find objectionable. Value judgements therefore make the term one to use with care.

DEPENDENT PERSONALITY FEATURES

These people show marked dependent traits, to their parents, spouses, doctors, hospitals, drug treatment, etc. They are people who easily become 'addicted' to drugs and doctors.

METHODS OF INVESTIGATIONS

The clinical way of assessing personality features has already been discussed. It is essentially that of the biographer. First class writers have the ability to sketch a personality bringing it to life in a few paragraphs; students might try to emulate this when they describe their patients.

Many psychiatrists in describing personality use concepts of emotional growth—from immaturity to maturity. In this context, one guide to 'maturity' lies in the patient's psychosexual development and present sexual life.

MANAGEMENT AND TREATMENT

(1) It has been emphasized that the presence of one or some of the personality features described does not imply that the patient is psychiatrically ill.

(2) It is useful to have some notion of 'stress threshold'. Everyone at a certain level of stress will develop psychiatric symptoms such as anxiety and depression. People with the features described above tend to have a low 'stress' tolerance and they react to stress with symptoms that are an exaggeration of their main personality features. Management here depends on outlining the 'stress' and modifying this or the patient's reaction to it.

(3) The development of 'depressive illness' (whether reactive or endogenous—see chapter 12) in patients with the personality features mentioned can produce an accentuation of these features, e.g. obsessional symptoms developing in an obsessional person—hysterical symptoms developing in an hysterical personality. The actual depressive symptoms *can be overlooked unless they are specifically asked for.* This is important as treatment with anti-depressive medication may be of great value therapeutically.

(4) Radical alterations in personality structure are probably not possible; psychoanalysis would be the only treatment that might claim to effect this.

SUMMARY

The meaning of the word 'personality' is discussed. The psychologist's measures of personality are useful in research, but not in clinical work.

Certain common personality features are outlined.

Suggestions are made about the significance of psychiatric symptoms developing in these personalities. The importance of depressive illness in this regard is emphasized.

REFERENCES

Eysenck, H. J., *Sense and Nonsense in Psychology*. Pelican (Harmondsworth, 1972). A very readable account of a psychologist's approach to personality structure and other related subjects.

Chodoff, P. and Lyons, H., 'Hysteria and the hysterical personality', *Am. J. Psychiat.*, 114: 734-40 (1958). An account of the hysterical personality.

7

HISTORY TAKING

INTRODUCTION

In psychiatry, as in all branches of medicine, a carefully taken history is of the greatest importance. Students should recognize that certain differences exist between history taking in psychiatry and medicine:

(1) While it is necessary that the presenting symptoms and their development should be clearly detailed, something other than a 'fact finding' history is needed. The patient must also be 'understood'—in a biographical sense—as a person. *A method of history taking that concentrates on fact finding can hinder the understanding aspects of the interview.*

For the patient to give an account of his life history to an understanding person who is able to listen with a degree of detachment may enable the patient himself to gain a measure of detachment from his difficulties. History taking is thus a part of treatment, rather than a necessary formality before treatment proper begins. In this regard clinical clerking by students can, if properly done, be an important part of the patient's treatment.

(2) In assessing a psychiatric patient—his illness and his personality—it is usually essential to obtain information from sources other than the patient. The more severe the illness, the more necessary does this become. Usually the husband, wife, mother, father or nearest relative of the patient should be seen. Only rarely can the whole family situation be ignored in understanding the patient and his symptoms.

It is also sometimes necessary to obtain detailed information about the patient's behaviour at school or at work, and the facts so obtained may be helpful, not only for diagnosis but also in planning the patient's management after he leaves hospital. This sort of information is often obtained for the doctor by a psychiatric social worker.

(3) In addition, regular interviews are the setting for treatment in psychiatry. This may be:

(a) on a supportive basis, or

(b) where the interview situation itself becomes a therapeutic mechanism which is intended to produce beneficial changes in the patient.

Both these types of interview situations can be called *psychotherapy,* but this term is often restricted to (b).

These three aspects of psychiatric history taking often puzzle students, who are used to taking a history from the patient only, on a question and answer basis.

Other problems also arise in psychiatric history taking. Psychiatric patients often can provoke a mixture of feelings in students—pity, sympathy, amusement, contempt, hostility, anger, fear are common. Patients, too, may be hostile or affectionate to the student and he must learn to accept this without either getting angry or too friendly or attached to the patient. What is needed is a detached but understanding and accepting attitude. Such an attitude is particularly difficult to maintain if the student himself, or someone in his family, has symptoms or difficulties similar to those which the patient reports. The student should learn to recognize problems arising from his own attitudes and discuss them with one of his tutors.

The difficulties and complexities of the psychiatric interview situation can be reduced by discussing it under the following headings:

(1) history taking from a new patient

(2) the principles of *supportive care*. Supportive care is of the utmost importance in all branches of medicine and is the cornerstone of general medical and psychiatric practice (chapter 9).

(3) the principles that underlie *psychotherapy proper* (chapter 11).

HISTORY TAKING FROM A NEW PATIENT

Ordinary history taking in psychiatry has two aims:

(1) *To Detail the Main Complaints*

The development and possible causes of the main symptoms must be detailed, and it is important to find how they have interfered with the patient's life in all its aspects.

The patient's 'physical' and 'mental' state are then defined, and usually it will then be possible to 'diagnose' the patient's symptoms, i.e., classify them into one or other of the diagnostic groupings already discussed.

(2) *To obtain a Biographical Understanding of the Patient as a Person*

In particular one should try and imagine oneself in the patient's everyday life, at work and at home, and then try to picture the world as the patient experiences it.

As has been mentioned a method of history taking that concentrates on symptoms can make an understanding of the patient difficult.

Psychiatric history taking cannot be rushed, and it is often the first stage in treatment. Adequate time should therefore be allowed for the initial history taking—*at least* an hour. Students should introduce themselves to the patient by name, and should see that both they and the patient are comfortably seated. Note taking should be as unobtrusive as possible. It is useful for students to have a scheme for case taking available (see appendix 1).

The student's main role in psychiatric history taking should be that of *an interested listener*. The patient will however need guiding

31

along the main paths of history taking, though the extent of this will vary from patient to patient. Missing details can always be sought after the patient has been encouraged to give his own account with only occasional prompting. Students must learn how to encourage the patient to give a history with minimal questioning and interruptions.

Reason for Referral

It is most important to get a clear account of why the patient has come for help at this time, who referred him and for what reasons.

Presenting Symptoms

'How long have you been ill?' 'What are your main complaints?' After a few opening questions the patient should be allowed to describe his symptoms in his own way, without interruption. What he emphasizes or, equally, what he leaves out at this stage may help in understanding the patient. How did the symptoms begin, and how have they interfered with his work, his home life, his relations with other people and recreations? It is useful here for the student to ask the patient to describe a typical day in his life and to say how the symptoms have interfered with what he regards as his normal pattern.

Have there been similar symptoms before? Has anyone in the family had similar symptoms and has the patient ever known anyone with similar problems? How does the patient explain his symptoms—what does he think they are due to—what is he frightened they mean?

These are the sort of questions that need answering, but the way they are asked, and the time they are asked will vary from patient to patient. Students can only learn this by practice, and by seeing more experienced people talking to patients. As in medicine and surgery, leading questions should be avoided.

Biography

The biographical aspects of history taking should then be started—usually by asking the patient where he was born, and about his family. Here questions should not be just 'How old are your parents?' or 'What did they die of?', but the patient should *be encouraged to talk about his parents as people* and to describe the family situation when he was a child. The way he describes his parents, siblings, his school, his school friends, will give valuable clues in assessing the patient's personality make up.

The patient should be encouraged to describe his school days, his work history, courtship, marriage and present family life. At the first interview it is usually not necessary or desirable to probe deeply into the patient's sexual life, but if problems in this field are presented by the patient, or if they seem specially relevant, students must learn how to ask the necessary intimate questions openly and frankly.

32

PERSONALITY

An attempt should be made to understand the patient's *personality*. Often valuable information about this comes from the patient's relatives, but the patient should be asked 'tell me what sort of a person you were before you became ill'. Important personality features met with in psychiatric patients have been described in chapter 6.

PREVIOUS HEALTH

The patient's *previous physical and mental health* needs to be asked about in detail. Accurate information will be needed about this, so that if the patient has previously been in hospital, a summary from the hospital can be obtained. Previous psychiatric illnesses are often similar to the present symptoms and response to previous treatment is a valuable guide to present management.

MENTAL STATE

Students find that describing the mental state of a patient is a difficult task. This is because it *is* difficult to describe behaviour and feelings, and because students are unfamiliar with psychiatric illness. The separation of *history* from the *mental state* is important. *The mental state is an assessment of what is actually going on in the patient's mental life at the time of the interview. The history is an account of the development of the symptoms and the changes in behaviour that led to referral.*

General Appearance and Behaviour

From the time the student first meets the patient, and all the time the history is being taken, the student should be *observing* the patient. He should notice the patient's general appearance, the mode of dressing, general cleanliness, evidence of weight loss. Is the patient co-operative, is he in touch with his surroundings? Is he slow in his movements and speech (retardation)? Is he restless (agitation)?

Patients vary from the very co-operative and intelligent, to the stuporous and non-responding. It is important that students should learn how to describe the patient's general behaviour in an accurate way.

Talk

The *form* of the patient's talk must be described. Does he say much or little? Is his talk slow or fast? Is it coherent or discursive? Are there sudden silences or changes of topic? Are strange associations or words used?

Mood

The patient's mood is then described—the patient should be asked, 'How do you feel in yourself?' 'How are your spirits?' or similar questions. Many varieties of mood may be present—not merely happiness or sadness. There is also anxiety, irritability, suspicion, fear and excitement. The changes that are observed in the mood are important and note should be taken of what appears to influence it. Are the patient's talk and preoccupations appropriate to the mood?

Thought Content

The patient's main *preoccupations* must be noted. What does he worry about? Is this all day or only at night? Are there suicidal thoughts? ('Have you felt that life is not worth living?') More abnormal features must be specifically asked about if clinically relevant. The main abnormalities are:

1. *Delusions and Misinterpretations*

What is the patient's attitude to his environment and people around him? Does he misinterpret any happenings? Does he think anyone treats him in a special way or persecutes him or influences him in any way? Do people seem to laugh at him? shun him? Do they try and harm him or annoy him? Does he think he is at fault in any way?

Delusions are false beliefs that cannot be altered by reasoning with the patient. In general they are either delusions of grandeur, poverty, persecution, self reproach, or hypochondriacal in content.

2. *Hallucinations*

Auditory, visual, olfactory, gustatory, tactile, somatic hallucinations should be clearly defined if present. Do they occur at night only, or in company with other people? What is the content of the auditory hallucinations?

Some patients complain of feelings of unreality, as if they have changed, and their actions feel automatic. This symptom is known as *depersonalization*. When the outside world appears different the symptom is termed *derealization*.

3. *Obsessional Features*

Obsessional thoughts and impulses should be asked about (see chapter 10). Does he recognize their inappropriateness? Does he repeat actions such as hand washing?

4. *Phobic Symptoms* (see chapter 10)

Orientation, Memory, Intelligence, Attention and Concentration

The patient's general intelligence can be assessed from the history, school and work record. The patient's memory can be assessed from the history and its correlation with that given by the relatives. If abnormalities are thought to be present then a detailed methodical examination needs to be carried out (see chapter 16).

Is the patient correctly orientated to time and place? Does he remember recent events clearly? This is an important part of the examination, particularly in the general hospital wards, when disturbed behaviour is often associated with clouding of consciousness. Can the patient concentrate or is he easily preoccupied?

Insight and Judgment

How does the patient regard his present state? Does he think he is ill? If so, what does he think is wrong? Does he think he will get well?

PHYSICAL EXAMINATION

Unless the patient has been referred from a physician and has recently had a full medical examination, all patients should be examined physically. In particular, relevant physical abnormalities should be looked for specifically, e.g., peripheral neuritis and evidence of liver disease in alcoholics; focal neurological abnormalities in dementing patients and so on.

HISTORY FROM INFORMANTS

It has been emphasized that it is usually essential to obtain an independent history from the person closest to the patient. This is usually the wife or husband, mother, father or children. It is often helpful and of interest to obtain the stories of a number of relatives so that a 'total' picture of the patient and his illness can be obtained. Again relatives should be allowed to describe the patient as a person before the illness began, to describe how the symptoms seem to have developed and how they have interfered with the patient's life.

Students should realize that, by the time the patient comes for treatment, relatives will have become 'involved' to varying extents with the patient's symptoms. Most relatives can appreciate and be sympathetic towards someone in their family with pain or shortness of breath. Psychiatric symptoms such as irritability, depression or anxiety are not so easily accepted by relatives. Their basis is not understood and patients are expected to be able to 'pull themselves out of it'. Relatives become involved with the symptoms and react according to their own personality make-up in various ways, e.g. the wife of an alcoholic has quite different problems to deal with from the wife of a patient with hypertension.

The involvement of the patient and his symptoms with the whole family should bring to the attention of the student that the family is the basic unit in our society and *in psychiatry the whole family needs to be considered*. Often more than one member is affected, e.g., the influence of an anxious phobic mother on the development of her children is easily observed. These family interactions are of the greatest interest, and provide for the psychiatrist one of the continuing interests in his daily work. 'Why, for instance, did this patient become alcoholic when his parents were so strictly "teetotal", and why does his wife become depressed when he stops drinking?' 'Why has their eldest daughter left home and why does the youngest son have a peptic ulcer?'

These sorts of family findings are not uncommon, and in their limited time of psychiatric clerking students should endeavour to see their patient's spouses, parents and children in order to appreciate more of these problems.

Psychiatry history taking as presented here sounds a formidable and time consuming operation. Students should, however, learn to take such a history from a new day or outpatient in 60-90 minutes, while 30-45 minutes should be spent with the appropriate relatives. For inpatients the history should be taken in more detail. It is often best to do this in two interviews of about an hour each. In addition relatives must be seen in every case and a full physical examination of the patient made. He should then try to assemble all the information he has obtained in some sort of relevant clinical manner—a *psychiatric formulation*.

SUMMARY

A good history is the cornerstone of clinical psychiatry.

It has a diagnostic and an understanding function. Differences between a typical medical and psychiatric history are discussed.

A method of history taking is outlined.

The value of a history from the nearest relatives is emphasized.

The student should recognize that to fully understand his patients he will need to spend time with them and to show real concern and interest. He must learn to be accepting and to exclude his own personal set of values from the transaction with the patient.

8

PSYCHIATRIC FORMULATION

Psychiatric diagnosis is essentially a way of grouping symptoms and signs into certain groups of 'illness'. The exercise of applying these labels is important, but it does not have the relevance that it has in general medicine or surgery. There the treatment and prognosis often almost automatically follows once the diagnosis has been firmly established. In psychiatry there are many important variables that need to be considered, as well as the diagnosis, and this information should be assembled as a 'psychiatric formulation'.

In a psychiatric formulation *relevant* facts (*not a repeat of the history*) are presented in a *significant* rather than formal order, and these facts then discussed from the point of view of:

(1) Diagnosis
(2) Aetiology
(3) Further investigations
(4) Treatment
(5) Prognosis

Psychiatric formulation is an essential part of the training of psychiatrists; but medical students should try and consider psychiatric problems in this way. Because of lack of experience their main problem will be in assessing what is and what is not clinically relevant.

Two examples will indicate the sort of formulation that students should be able to master by the end of their period of clinical clerking.

Example 1

Mrs B. aged 70 has had severe depressive symptoms for about 3 months that seem to have come on without any precipitating factors in her social or personal life. There was a previous 'nervous breakdown' when she was 21 at the time of a broken engagement, and she remembers sleeping badly and being unduly tired at that time. One of her brothers committed suicide. Now she is agitated, sleeping badly and has suicidal ideas. She is correctly orientated but her answers to questions about current events are impaired. She lives with her husband in their own home.

Diagnosis: Depressive illness.

Aetiology: No precipitating factors known, but there is a history of a previous attack. There is also a likely family history of depressive illness.

Further investigations: It will be useful to fully assess her memory functions—and particularly to note her answers to simple questions on current political events. It is likely however that this impairment of cognitive function is a consequence of the depressive illness, and does not indicate the presence of a dementing process, as she finds it difficult to concentrate and is agitated.

Treatment: In view of the severity of the depression, its short course, and the presence of suicidal ideas, a course of E.C.T. is likely to produce improvement in the shortest time. It will be best to admit her to hospital to arrange for this. Alternatively, she could be admitted to hospital and given anti-depressive medication.

Prognosis: Good for present illness; but a further attack may occur.

Example 2

Mr M. aet. 24 years, a welder, came to out-patients with headaches and indigestion for 2 years. The headaches are uncomfortable and he has recognized that they are provoked by him becoming angry at work or at home. His 'indigestion' describes the occurrence of epigastric pains that are made worse by eating but relieved by alkalis. He has had months without these pains, but the headaches have been fairly persistent over the last 2 years. It is significant that he says he is a worrier and has always been nervous since childhood. His father left his mother when the patient was 10 and has not been seen since. The patient, one sister and his mother had a difficult time financially after this. His mother is a 'nervous' person, who always has a headache, and one of her brothers has a duodenal ulcer. Two years ago, he married; he has 2 children. The marriage is described as 'good' but there are frequent rows. At work 'the foreman always picks on me because I am the youngest! I get angry and give as good as he gives'.

On examination he was an anxious, tense young man, who smoked constantly throughout the interview. There is no physical abnormality other than epigastric tenderness.

Diagnosis: Probable peptic ulceration. Headaches and general anxiety symptoms.

Aetiology: His childhood had obvious difficulties and further interviews would help to clarify these and his personality structure. There is a family history of peptic ulceration.

Further investigations: Barium meal examination.

Treatment: Appropriate diet and alkali treatment is indicated for the indigestion. He talks well and further interviews about his early life, and his present attitude to authority might be helpful. He might later benefit from treatment in a group situation.

Prognosis: His symptoms should improve but problems at home with wife and children may develop further and these will need to be observed.

SUMMARY

In a psychiatric formulation, relevant facts are arranged so that the clinical problem can be discussed from the point of view of differential diagnosis, aetiology, further investigation, treatment and prognosis.

9

SUPPORTIVE CARE

In their training, students get little experience of the sort of doctor-patient interaction that is the cornerstone of medical practice and may be called *supportive care.*

This type of care is necessary for patients with chronic illnesses or for patients who have recurring attacks of symptoms. Such patients are the rule in general medical and psychiatric practice. Supportive care is the mainstay of general practitioners' treatment.

In all branches of medicine, the basis of supportive care is the doctor's interest in his patient. For the patient to be able to rely on seeing the same interested doctor at regular intervals is of great help, even if, to an outsider, nothing very eventful appears to happen at these meetings. In general, doctors who are more interested in the person with the illness rather than in the illness itself are usually the most successful in supportive care.

In seeing psychiatric patients regularly in a supportive situation it is important that the patient is given an adequate time for his appointment. In addition to these regular appointments the doctor should be willing to see the patient at other times, and should develop the ability of seeming unhurried, even if the interview has to be a short one.

INTERESTED LISTENING

In supportive care the doctor adopts the role of an interested, sympathetic and accepting listener. At interview, the patient usually talks about his symptoms at first, but most patients move on to talk about their particular problems at work or at home. The acceptance and understanding of the doctor in dealing with these problems is of great benefit to the patient. Some psychiatric patients, unless stopped, will only talk about their symptoms (which are usually multiple). Such patients must be actively discouraged from doing this and should be encouraged to talk more about their particular interpersonal problems at work and at home. To give the patient an opportunity to ventilate, discuss and share his problems helps him to achieve a greater degree of detachment and objectivity, and makes it easier for him to find a solution himself. Generally patients are only too willing to talk about themselves and their problems. Sometimes they need encouragement, such as might be given by indicating that you regard what the patient is saying as important and that you are willing to listen.

39

REASSURANCE

This is an important part of the doctor's work, but should be offered with discrimination. If given prematurely it may discourage the patient from ventilating his problem fully and can erect a barrier between doctor and patient by conveying the impression that the doctor does not really understand just how ill the patient feels. Simply to rely on the passage of time or the administration of drugs and to reinforce this with suggestions that the patient will recover from his symptoms is unwise, as the only result may be loss of confidence in the doctor when the predicted outcome does not ensue. In particular, reassurance will be of little or no value in depressed patients who have hypochondriacal symptoms unless adequate treatment is first initiated to correct the mood disorder.

When the patient is worried about the probability of a physical ill-ness as the cause of his symptoms, it is, of course, important to re-assure him that he is physically well, but only after any necessary examinations and tests have been carried out. Other patients may not be worried about the possibility of having cancer or heart disease but fear they might be 'going mad', and 'have to be certified' or that they might 'lose control' of themselves, or harm someone else. When pos-sible, reassurance here can be helpful to the patient in allaying his fears but it must be followed by a search for the cause of the fear and its adequate treatment in the same way that reassurance about the absence of physical disease must be followed by an inquiry into the emotional causes of the symptoms.

EXPLANATION

Explanation that symptoms such as palpitation or headache are due to anxiety and not to heart or brain disease may accompany reassur-ance. The doctor needs to remember that his preferred explanations may be more reassuring to himself than to the patient. Explanations in anatomical and physiological terms, though impressing the patient with the doctor's learning, may not mean anything more than that, unless the explanation falls within the scope of the patient's own knowledge and experience. It is more useful to draw on your know-ledge of the patient's past history than to explain symptoms in terms of hypothetical forces, e.g. 'You recall that you had palpitations on the day of an important examination.' Explanation in psychopatho-logical terms like those used by psychiatrists to discuss between them-selves their own formulations are worse than useless and, if they serve any function at all, it is only as a means of intellectualizing the prob-lem and making it more difficult to deal with.

Use only every-day language which the patient understands and, if possible, his own terms.

40

ADVICE

There are times when the doctor should properly offer advice, and to withhold it would be for him to fail in his duty; but there are other occasions when to give advice is extremely hazardous. Generally speaking, advice must be given when the doctor knows from his medical training that certain things are important in the treatment of the patient's illness but, even here, it is often wiser to explain to the patient *why* certain things are important. When the matter is not a technical one in which the doctor's medical skill and knowledge are appropriate, but one which concerns the patient's personal life, any advice the doctor gives is likely to reflect his own private experiences or beliefs. Such advice may be better withheld. The various ways in which the patient might approach his problem and the possible consequences of doing this can be discussed instead. Often doctors give inappropriate advice. An example would be the recommendation given to a woman to have children, when her underlying problem, one of doubt about her ability to function adequately as a mother, is largely unresolved. Frequently the doctor's advice relates to what he himself would do in the circumstances, but it is important to remember that the patient has not the doctor's personality and resources, and in any case the doctor is not in the same position as the patient and does not necessarily see things in the way the patient does.

Allow the patient time to talk about his problems fully, explore them with him, and then suggest that he might like to think things over and see how he feels in a few days; perhaps he would like to talk about it again or let you know next time what he decides to do.

MANIPULATION OF THE ENVIRONMENT

It is sometimes difficult for the doctor to decide when to attempt to manipulate the patient's environment. In these days of social service benefits, insurance against sickness and for many other purposes, patients frequently ask for certificates and reports and giving these is often part of the doctor's work; but how far should the doctor go, and when? Should he ring the employer, talk to the wife or husband, order a holiday or a change of job, make representations to government departments or social service agencies? Increasingly doctors are asked to do some or all of these things.

In general, the more ill the patient, the more it is important to help in this way, e.g. the chronic schizophrenic patient may need help with his job, or need to have his illness discussed with relatives and the likely consequences explained. The less ill patient, whose neurosis and emotional disturbance leave him more able to cope with his environment himself, may well be encouraged to look at the difficulties he experiences in doing these things for himself. At times, however, the patient 'needs' the doctor's permission: for example, to take a holiday.

Social, domestic and economic problems may aggravate a psychological illness and it may be very important for the doctor to take them into account. In hospitals, social workers offer valuable help and are usually well versed in the community services and facilities available to the patient. In private practice, the doctor may be able to refer the patient to a hospital or to an appropriate social service agency and he should make himself acquainted with the resources available in his area and use them when the patient's interest requires it. Many patients may not be aware of their rights regarding unemployment and social service benefits and other forms of help which are available to them.

Although patients should be encouraged to deal with these problems themselves, there are occasions when they should not take any steps, especially in matters which may have important consequences, until they have recovered from their illness sufficiently to appreciate the significance of their decisions. Depressed patients often find many problems in their social environment which are either not present or seem trivial when they recover, and for which the action they would have taken while ill would have been unnecessary or undesirable.

DEPENDENCE

Most young doctors are worried by the prospect of patients becoming too dependent on them. It is true that some patients do make heavy demands on their doctors and seem to be unable to get along without continual support.

It is necessary to remember that patients are, in reality, very dependent on doctors for understanding and treatment and that doctors are also dependent on patients for the continued practice of their profession and hence, directly or indirectly, their livelihood. Having recognized this, we are in a better position to assess the interaction between doctor and patient in respect of dependency needs. Patients with neurotic illness are likely to have a greater need than most people for a dependent relationship and they may also be more sensitive to rejection, or other attitudes on the part of the doctor which arouse emotional responses. The patient's irrational attitudes to, and expectations of, the doctor are part of the neurotic illness and need to be recognized and treated as such.

This is quite a complex problem, but the doctor can best deal with it by being aware of his own responses to difficult patients. When students feel themselves angry or upset with a particular patient, they should think about all the circumstances of the case. Such limited excursions into self-analysis may be helpful. It is essential to recognize just what the patient wants from the doctor and this may be different from what the patient asks for, as the real need may be either intentionally or unconsciously concealed. When it is made clear what the patient does want, bringing it out into the open and discussing it frankly may go a long way towards resolving undue dependence.

If you are unable to recognize or deal with the causes of a patient's dependence it may be necessary to accept these needs for a dependent relationship and give the patient some time to discuss his problems at regular intervals, perhaps weekly, fortnightly, monthly or at even longer periods. Continued interest in the nature and the meaning of the dependence may enable its meaning eventually to become clearer and so permit it to be dealt with.

DRUG TREATMENT

Drug administration is usually an important part of supportive care. For patients who have been in hospital with schizophrenia, drug treatment may have to go on indefinitely and the patient and his relatives must constantly be reminded of the importance of his taking tablets. Depressed patients may need medication for several months before the tablets are reduced gradually.

More difficult is the more frequently encountered patient with mixed neurotic symptoms. Sometimes anxiety is predominant, at other times headache, or sleeplessness or depression or premenstrual symptoms. There are now available many active but potentially dangerous drugs for the symptomatic treatment of anxiety, headache, sleeplessness, etc., and it is easier to write a prescription for these than to try to help the patient by psychological or social means. However, many investigations have shown that these are the sorts of patients who improve symptomatically on chemically inactive 'placebos'. This important clinical problem is discussed further in chapters 10 and 21.

THE FAMILY

In concluding these notes on supportive care, it is important to remember the family as a whole. Often it is helpful to see the patient and his parent or spouse regularly and so 'spread the support' more widely than the patient alone.

Gradually doctors should 'wean' the patients from attending by lengthening the time between interviews—then at the appropriate time saying: 'Well, I won't give you another appointment but I shall always be pleased to see you again if you have any problems or your symptoms come back'.

CARE OF PATIENTS WITH NEUROSIS IN GENERAL PRACTICE

One of the general practitioner's main tasks in present-day medical practice is to treat patients with neurotic symptoms. The following comments deal with three aspects of the management of these patients.

1. The Attitude of the Doctor to Psychiatric Problems

The way the doctor deals with psychiatric problems depends upon his own personality characteristics and the attitude he developed towards psychiatric patients in his medical training. In the past this latter was often not helpful. Students now get some experience of clinical clerking on psychiatric patients, they see something of individual and group psychotherapy and their attitudes to psychiatric illness are brought to their notice by their tutors. When they enter practice they should be in a better position to manage psychiatric problems than their predecessors.

The doctor, on the one hand, may have similar emotional problems to the patient, and he may identify with the patient and become deeply involved with the patient's problem. On the other hand, the doctor may be intolerant of emotional problems. He may thoroughly investigate the patient from a physical point of view, and finding no physical abnormality reject the patient as 'functional', 'neurotic', unimportant or trivial, and do nothing to help the patient's emotional problems.

The doctor should be able to accept emotional problems as real and important; as real as appendicitis or bronchitis, yet remain objective but accepting of the patient's problems.

2. The Anxious Patient

Usually the anxious patient comes complaining of physical symptoms—headaches, indigestion, fatigue, vague aches and pains. These symptoms are often expressions of dissatisfaction, anger, frustration and discontent. If the doctor accepts the physical complaints as *the illness,* the chances of understanding the underlying causes are diminished. If a thorough physical examination shows no abnormality, then investigations should be limited. Repeated investigations of symptoms and different symptomatic remedies with later specialist referrals (to reassure the general practitioner) are not the best ways of treating these patients; neither is the symptomatic treatment of these patients with drugs without attempts to discover the causes of the symptoms. Doctors must be prepared to listen to these patients and move from the symptoms to the patient as a person and discover the *meaning of the anxiety symptoms.* Time must be given so that a full psychiatric history is taken; then the principles of supportive care previously described applied.

3. The Chronic Neurotic Patient

Many general practitioners find these patients tiresome with their chronic multiple complaints. It is best if they are seen for regular but brief interviews (say 15 minutes). They should be allowed to talk freely and it has been mentioned that patients should not be encouraged to talk about physical or psychiatric symptoms but helped to talk about interpersonal difficulties and feelings. Patients seeing the doctor regularly, become dependent upon him, but may be able to function fairly well at home and at work because of this regular medical help. The doctor's acceptance of the patient's difficulties helps the patient to cope with his problems. It is however important that the doctor should not encourage dependence and should, if possible, aim gradually to wean the patient from medical attention.

SUMMARY

The importance of supportive care for psychiatric patients in general medical practice is emphasized. The main ingredients are the doctor's interest in his patient and the patient's faith in the doctor. The patient must be given time to talk about his problems. Reassurance, explanation, advice, social changes and drug administration are discussed. The doctor's own attitudes to psychiatric problems are commented on in more detail.

REFERENCE

Balint, M., *The Doctor, his Patient and the Illness.* 2nd ed., Pitman (London, 1964). This book reviews the problems that general practitioners have with psychiatric illness.

10

NEUROSIS

Neurotic symptoms are among the commonest groups of symptoms that doctors meet with in clinical work. It is important therefore, that students should be able to recognize these symptoms, understand something about their production, and learn certain principles that will guide them in treating neurotic patients.

Neurotic illnesses are characterized by the presence of various somatic and mental symptoms as well as disturbances in the social adjustment of the individual. Clinical judgement about 'social adjustment' depends on a consideration of the patient's interpersonal relationships, and his capacity for enjoyment and work achievement. There is no yardstick for diagnosing neurosis other than the observer's knowledge and clinical experience, hence the reliability of the diagnosis 'neurosis' is not high, even among psychiatrists.

AETIOLOGY

Three general groups of factors are important in considering the aetiology of the neuroses:

Genetic and constitutional factors have an important effect in moulding personality structure.

Personality patterns developed in early childhood: experiences at certain stages of emotional development have a lasting effect on later personality.

Present day problems of every conceivable sort.

Though some schools of psychiatry emphasize one or other of these factors, they are all important in every patient. From the point of view of treatment, knowledge of present day problems is of particular importance.

PSYCHOPATHOLOGY

As has been mentioned in chapter 5 the most valuable explanations of neurotic symptoms and neurotic personality structure are to be found in psychodynamic theories. The symptoms are considered to be the visible signs of unconscious conflicts and theoretically a 'cure' can only occur if these conflicts are resolved. Central to such theories is the concept that neurotic symptoms are the unsuccessful attempts by the personality to deal with anxiety. *Neurotic symptoms are not conscious or feigned or deliberate in any way. It is important that students should recognize this.*

History taking will show that these patients have usually had neurotic symptoms in childhood—anxiety, phobias, feeding problems, temper tantrums, shyness, enuresis. The present day problems that precipitate neurotic symptoms typically involve hostility, sexuality or dependency. Because of personality structure these emotions cannot be expressed directly and are distorted or repressed. The resultant anxiety may be experienced as *generalized anxiety* or in some cases as *phobic* symptoms where the anxiety is felt only in specific situations. In other patients (according to psychopathological theories) anxiety is 'converted' into hysterical symptoms, while in others anxiety is 'controlled' by obsessional symptoms.

Age and Sex Incidence

Neurotic symptoms are more frequent in women. They may occur at any age, but most neurotic patients are between 15 and 50.

SYMPTOMS AND SIGNS

Neurotic symptoms can be subdivided into a number of groupings:

- (1) Anxiety symptoms
- (2) Depressive symptoms
- (3) Obsessional symptoms
- (4) Hysterical symptoms

Some neurotic patients have symptoms confined mainly to one of the above groups of symptoms. In other patients symptoms may be present from two, three or four of the above groupings. When all four groups of symptoms are present the condition is often called a *'mixed neurotic reaction'*. To simplify description these four groups of symptoms will be dealt with separately.

ANXIETY SYMPTOMS

The patient with generalized anxiety will complain of palpitations, tightness in the chest, headache, loss of appetite, sleeplessness, facial flushes, sweating, dizziness, tremulousness, and undue fatigue on physical or mental exertion. He is tense, apprehensive and a worrier, often concerned about his health. The somatic symptoms of which the patient complains are explainable as accompaniments of changes in functioning of the autonomic nervous system (predominantly sympathetic stimulation).

Some patients in addition to these general anxiety symptoms have more specific symptoms related to a particular situation, or to a particular object. Faintness, fatigue, palpitation, sweating, nausea and a sense of impending collapse are the main symptoms of these 'localized' anxiety or *phobic* symptoms. Gradually these phobic patients avoid the situations or objects that provoke the symptoms. e.g., the 'housebound housewife' who stays at home because the symptoms develop if she leaves the house on her own.

47

DEPRESSIVE SYMPTOMS

These are described in detail in chapter 12. The syndrome of *reactive depression* is probably the most frequently diagnosed neurotic group of symptoms. Again it is important to recognize that the patient usually presents with somatic complaints, i.e., sleep disturbance, anorexia, tiredness, weight loss, constipation, etc.

OBSESSIONAL SYMPTOMS

The characteristic feature of obsessional symptoms is that along with some mental happening, there is *an experience of subjective compulsion and of a resistance to it*. The mental happenings are:

(1) *Ideas or images, or phrases* (often obscene) that return to the patient's mind, though there is a subjective feeling of resistance to these ideas.

(2) *Impulses.* These are often aggressive in character—the patient may feel the urge to injure her child or attack people in the street. Again there is the sense of resistance to these impulses, but the impulse keeps returning to the patient's mind causing distress. It is important to recognize the obsessional nature of these impulses and to reassure the patient that she will *never* carry out these impulses.

(3) *Ruminations.* Here endless questionings return to the patient's mind usually about 'non-answerable' questions such as what is the meaning of life, and death, etc. Any event can lead the patient to return to these ruminations which he cannot stop.

In some neurotic patients obsessional symptoms are the predominant features, and the condition is then called *obsessive-compulsive neurosis.* This is one of the most crippling and distressing forms of psychiatric illness. In these patients, compulsive acts accompany the obsessional thinking, e.g., a patient has obsessional ideas that his hands are not clean and he will consequently transmit a disease to others. He therefore washes them several times, but the ideas return and he has to rewash his hands, though part of his mind recognizes it is unnecessary. If he tries not to wash his hands, he becomes extremely anxious and agitated and this is only relieved by further hand washing. In severe cases this repetitive hand washing may occupy the patient's whole day.

Obsessional symptoms are frequent in depressive illness; they can be prominent in some patients who have had an attack of encephalitis. They are occasionally seen in patients with a schizophrenic illness.

HYSTERICAL SYMPTOMS

The use of the word *hysteria* is a controversial one in psychiatry today. It should be used in one of two ways:

(1) To describe a certain type of personality (described in chapter 6), or

(2) To describe certain *symptoms* which are known as hysterical 'con-

version' symptoms. These symptoms, e.g. aphonia or weakness of a limb, are thought to be symbolic resolutions of emotional conflicts. *These 'motor' conversion symptoms only involve structures innervated by the voluntary nervous system* (compare anxiety symptoms). Psychopathological theories usually view the symptoms as a defence against anxiety (*primary gain*); but there is usually *secondary gain* when the symptoms are used for the patient's benefit (e.g. to receive attention and sympathy in the *sick role*), though the patient is not clearly conscious of the motive. This gain often seems perverse to others, but it may represent some satisfaction to the patient.

Hysterical symptoms can be:

(a) *Motor*

There is paralysis or weakness of any voluntary action (*not* individual muscle groups).

Abnormal movements—contractures, clonic or choreiform movements, torticollis are *sometimes* hysterical. They are more often due to organic lesions in the central nervous system.

Hysterical 'fits' occur in the presence of others, with manifest motivation and they usually have a theatrical quality. The sequence of an epileptic seizure does not occur (unless the patient is familiar with epilepsy). The patients do not injure themselves, bite their tongue, nor are they incontinent.

(b) *Sensory*

Anaesthetic areas of the skin are found that do not (usually) correspond to sensory nerve distribution. (Glove and stocking is the description of the usual distribution of the anaesthesia). Deafness, blindness, anosmia and loss of taste can also be hysterical symptoms. The problem of *pains* as hysterical symptoms is discussed in chapter 13. *In general, pains for which no physical basis can be found should NOT be labelled hysterical.*

(c) *Mental*

Amnesias and unusual mental states are the main ones; these last need only concern the psychiatrist. In hysterical amnesia the patient professes to have forgotten periods of his life; yet in his behaviour he shows none of the behavioural disturbances seen in patients with memory impairment, due to a chronic brain syndrome (chapter 15) e.g., he does not get lost, nor become neglectful of dress.

There are no 'signs or stigmata' of hysteria. Those recorded in the early literature on the subject were due to suggestion on the part of the examiner, and the ease with which these patients responded to the suggestion. Because of this, symptoms should not be suggested to the patient in history taking nor should physical examination be unnecessarily detailed (e.g., sensory examination of the central nervous system).

The use of the term hysteria to describe these symptoms presents several difficulties:

Follow up of patients labelled 'hysterical' has shown that a significant proportion of these patients develop definite organic disease (usually of the central nervous system) or schizophrenia or severe depression (sometimes with suicide). In such a follow up, a significant proportion of these patients were dead within a few years of the diagnosis of hysteria.

The use of the word hysteria has also been studied. Investigations have shown that the word 'hysteria' is used by doctors and non-medical people, as a reaction to frustrating and hostility provoking behaviour on the part of the particular patient—these are not reliable criteria on which to base a diagnosis.

Other errors in diagnosis are dependent on an exclusive preoccupation with *psychopathological theories* of hysteria.

The word *hysteria* should therefore be used:

(1) To describe patients who show the features of *the hysterical personality* (chapter 6). Their attention seeking behaviour can be called *histrionic*.

(2) To describe patients with conversion symptoms. *Students should use great caution in diagnosing hysterical conversion symptoms unless they are gross, occur in typical hysterical personalities and develop from an emotionally charged situation from which the symptoms will bring the patient some sort of gain.*

It is important to recognize that when people with hysterical personality features develop a physical or psychiatric illness (particularly neurological illnesses and depression) then hysterical symptoms can occur as *part* of the total clinical picture. It is important that the physical illness or depression is not missed because of the presence of the more obvious hysterical symptomatology.

Hysterical conversion reactions are by no means confined to patients with marked hysterical personality features; yet because the problems of positive diagnosis are complex, it should usually be left to a psychiatrist.

COMPENSATION CASES

The clinical problems here often involve the separation of hysterical and physical symptoms. These cases present complex clinical and social problems that require judgements from experienced clinicians.

It is important to recognize that any distinction between hysteria and malingering must be made from a clinical judgement of the patient's honesty and self knowledge—separation cannot be made by any tests. There is a paucity of follow-up studies in this area.

THE NATURAL HISTORY OF NEUROSIS

In most patients neurotic symptoms settle down within the course of a few months. In some patients symptoms are more disabling and long lasting. Long term follow up of this last group shows that there is a tendency for the symptoms to improve in time, irrespective of any treatment measure employed. *This fact makes the assessment of the value of treatment in neurosis a difficult problem.* Patients with anxiety and depressive symptoms will do best, patients with mainly obsessional symptoms worst.

DIAGNOSIS

Negative Aspects of the Diagnosis

Somatic symptoms, e.g., palpitations, headaches, anorexia, weight loss are common neurotic symptoms. Diagnosis of neurosis must therefore exclude a *relevant* organic cause for the symptoms.

In this regard there are two common clinical errors:

(1) The use of multiple investigations to 'exclude' physical disorders, when a complete history (including the psychiatric aspects) has not been taken. As will be mentioned later, the diagnosis of neurosis is often made at the end of a long series of investigations and specialist referrals. It is much easier to find the meaning of the symptoms when the patient first presents.

(2) In excluding a *relevant* organic cause for the symptoms it is important to recognize, for example, that 'mild hypertension' or anaemia, radiographic changes of spondylitis, or the presence of chronic sinusitis does not necessarily account for the symptoms complained of. The correct assessment of the relevance of physical abnormalities to the patient's complaints is one of the hallmarks of the competent physician or surgeon. It should be mentioned here that enthusiasm in treating such minor pathology in neurotic patients does little good.

Positive Aspects of the Diagnosis

Even if the physical examination and the relevant investigations are negative then the symptoms complained of are not necessarily neurotic. It is necessary to make a *positive* diagnosis of neurosis. In this regard the following features are important:

(1) *The developmental history*

The manner in which a neurotic patient describes parents, schooldays and relationships with other people is a characteristic clinical fact that students must learn by experience. The assessment of the patient's sexual development, present sexual life, work record and interests are all important in assessing the patient's personality structure and making a positive diagnosis of neurosis. The value of this assessment is dependent upon psychiatric experience.

(2) *Similar previous symptoms at times of 'stress'*

This is an important aspect of positive diagnosis. Such 'stress' may be impending marriage, death of parents or friends, change of jobs, operations, examinations, moving house, etc. Similar symptoms at these times are important points in making a positive diagnosis.

51

(3) *Relationship of symptoms to present problems*

It has been emphasized that in psychiatric history taking, the relationship of present symptoms to present interpersonal or social problems must be assessed in the context of an understanding of the patient's personality. This is the third important aspect of the positive diagnosis. Again this assessment is dependent on psychiatric experience.

UNCERTAIN DIAGNOSIS

Clinically there is an important group of patients who have symptoms that cannot be positively diagnosed as neurotic, yet no physical abnormalities are found to be present. Specialist referral may be helpful in establishing a diagnosis, but if not, and it remains uncertain, patients may need to be treated symptomatically and seen regularly to assess the physical or neurotic (or a combined) basis for the symptoms, by follow up over months (or years).

NEUROSIS AND PHYSICAL DISORDER

As will be emphasized in chapter 13 *physical illness and neurosis frequently occur together,* and diagnostic possibilities are not either/ or but often both. In these patients it is important to try and assess the extent to which disability is due to neurosis or physical causes and both may require treatment.

DIAGNOSIS WITHIN THE NEUROTIC SYNDROME

Of the various groups of neurotic symptoms described the depressive ones are the most important particularly because effective anti-depressive treatment is now available. Anxiety and depression are both disorders of mood and usually occur together. Depressive symptoms in a patient with an hysterical personality can be labelled hysteria by the inexperienced. Obsessional symptoms can be the presenting signs of a depressive illness particularly in the elderly (see chapter 12). Obsessional symptoms must be distinguished, by the feeling of subjective compulsion and immediate resistance, from delusions, hallucinations, ideas of reference and self reproach.

PREVENTION AND TREATMENT

Prevention

Neurosis is thought to have its roots in early life, but except for general statements about parent-child relationships little of specific preventive value can be said in this regard. Iatrogenic symptoms can be minimized and here the indiscriminate use of the sphygmomanometer, excessive investigations without adequate indications, the unnecessary prescription of bed rest, and unnecessary limitation of physical exercise need to be mentioned, as does the unwise use of psychotherapeutic techniques by the inexperienced.

Because neurotic patients frequently complain of aches and pains, unnecessary operations are not infrequently performed. In one study, 235 neurotic patients were followed up over 6 years. Two hundred had operations in this time—usually gynaecological or concerned with the nose and throat. In most cases the operations did not relieve symptoms. Persistent right-sided abdominal aching due to a spastic colon is not infrequently 'treated' by appendicectomy for 'chronic appendicitis'. Again, follow up shows that symptom relief is not usually permanent.

Treatment

Most neurotic symptoms respond well to supportive care at a general practitioner level. Psychiatric referral is needed in a minority of patients.

Time should be given for the initial interview and *adequate interested listening* should be the general approach. A full physical examination with reassurance and explanation of symptoms are important. The general practitioner should concentrate in further interviews on current problems and not probe deeply into the patient's past life or sexual history. The principles of supportive care in general practice have been described in chapter 9.

Drug Treatment in Neurosis

Drug treatment may play a valuable part in the general care of neurotic patients.

(1) *Anxious patients* often respond well to placebos, sedatives and tranquillizing drugs. It is not easy to assess the value of a specific drug for anxiety symptoms by a controlled trial. In a trial on anxious outpatients, two physicians with rather different attitudes to drug treatment found not only differing responses to the drugs, but also a different incidence of side-effects. Placebos relieve anxiety symptoms in a significant proportion of anxious patients. In controlled trials the dosage of the active drug used is crucial when tested against inert tablets. In one properly controlled trial Amytal 60 mg. and 120 mg. t.d.s. and phenobarbitone 15 mg. t.d.s. did not appreciably or consistently do better than inert tablets.

Diazepam (Valium) and other related benzodiazepines are today the anti-anxiety drugs of choice. They have been shown in controlled trials to be more effective than inert tablets. They are relatively safe if taken in overdosage. Only a small number of patients become physically dependent on them. They are perhaps best used by the patient when he feels anxious, or when he knows he will feel anxious rather than on a regular three times a day regime.

For patients with troublesome somatic symptoms of anxiety (e.g., palpitations) beta blocking drugs, e.g., propanolol 40mg., are being used.

In general, barbiturates should be avoided, because of dependency problems and the dangers from overdose. Diazepoxide drugs are superior in all respects.

(2) *The treatment of depressive symptoms* is described in chapter 12.

For patients with depressive and anxiety symptoms psychiatrists may use a combination of a monoamine oxidase inhibitor with a tranquillizing drug e.g. phenelzine (Nardil) 15 mg. t.d.s. and diazepam (Valium) 5 mg. t.d.s.

(3) *Obsessional symptoms* may be helped with anti-depressive or tranquillizing drugs, and it is important to decide clinically if anxiety and tension or depression is the predominant affect.

(4) *Hysterical symptoms* are not usually helped by drug treatment, unless they occur in the setting of a depressive illness.

Problems of Drug Treatment in Neurosis

(1) Drug treatment can be used too readily; it is better to spend more time listening to the patient.

(2) Because of the chronic nature of the symptoms, because drugs (barbiturates and amphetamines) are used that can produce dependence, and because of the patient's personality—*drug dependence* is a real problem.

(3) Suicide and attempted suicide are risks that should be kept in mind in prescribing drugs for all psychiatric patients. Drugs may need to be given only to a responsible relative, who will then give them to the patient daily.

(4) The biggest problem is the fluctuating and usually mild symptomatology and the increasing number of active (but potentially toxic) drugs available that can influence psychiatric symptoms. It has already been mentioned that placebos relieve neurotic symptoms in a significant proportion of patients and that drug dosage is crucial in trials of active substances for anxiety symptoms. Students are advised to learn how to use a small number of relatively safe drugs, and to use these, rather than each new preparation as it appears.

Psychiatric Referral

Certain patients with neurotic symptoms need to be referred to a psychiatrist for more specialized treatment than the average family doctor could be expected to provide. These patients are likely to be:

(1) Those with persistent anxiety, depressive, obsessional or hysterical symptoms. These patients have symptoms that have not responded to supportive care by the general practitioner, and interfere with the patient's life.

(2) Those with severe obsessional, phobic and hysterical symptoms, who are particularly resistant to treatment and for whom prolonged psychiatric treatment is usually needed.

The actual type of psychiatric treatment suggested for the individual neurotic patient, i.e. supportive care by the psychiatrist or drug treatment or individual or group psychotherapy, or behaviour therapy is a problem for the psychiatrist. Patients who might be suitable for psychotherapy are usually intelligent, young to middle-aged, who have persistent symptoms (usually anxiety), or long standing neurotic personality traits (perhaps with sexual problems). Social and economic factors are important in assessing referral to a psychotherapist, as usually psychotherapy is an expensive, long continued treatment.

ANOREXIA NERVOSA

Anorexia nervosa is a rare condition, but one that is seen regularly in the medical and psychiatric wards of general hospitals. It is an illness characterized by amenorrhoea and weight loss due to an elective restriction of food intake, because of morbid ideas about being fat. It is seen in adolescent girls. The amenorrhoea may precede the weight loss by several months. *'Anorexia' is usually a misnomer*, as these girls often have a good appetite—and may have episodes of overeating and of eating unusual things (e.g. mouldy bacon).

There will usually be found a poor premorbid sexual adjustment and a hostile relationship with the mother, who sometimes has an abnormal personality. There may be a history of childhood problems with food and conflicts with the mother over this.

Commonly there is no particular outside event that coincides with the onset of the symptoms. Other symptoms include restlessness, and the whole range of neurotic symptoms—depressive, anxiety, obsessional and hysterical. Patients are often interested in cooking and feeding others.

Aetiology

The illness can be considered as a phobic-avoidance response to the physical changes of puberty and their sexual and social implications.

Differential Diagnosis

Other wasting diseases of adolescence should be considered but the clinical syndrome of anorexia nervosa is a distinct one. Patients with hypopituitarism do not lose weight.

Course of Illness

This can be a chronic one and some patients die.

Treatment

In hospital, adequate nutrition should be given with fluid protein mixtures given as 'medicine'. Directives over eating rarely work for long. *Long term management* by one doctor (usually a psychiatrist) is needed. Problems of eating, as well as sexual and social adjustments, need attention over several years. Phenothiazines, e.g., chlorpromazine 100 mg. t.d.s., are often helpful in reducing restlessness and helping to put on weight. Insulin treatment can cause death.

SUMMARY

The main features of neurosis are described. The clinical features include combinations of anxiety, depressive, obsessional and hysterical symptoms.

The diagnosis should depend upon positive evidence of life long personality problems, previous symptoms at times of stress, and present interpersonal or social problems. Neurotic symptoms should not be attributed to minor physical abnormalities. Organic illness and neurotic symptoms frequently coexist.

Supportive care by the general practitioner with appropriate drug treatment will help most patients.

The G.P. needs to be interested and to give adequate time to these patients.

Suggestions are made about the sorts of patients who need psychiatric referral.

Anorexia nervosa is briefly described.

REFERENCES

Freud, S. (trans. Riviere, J.), *Introductory Lectures on Psychoanalysis*. 2nd ed., Allen & Unwin (London, 1961). Still the best introduction to Freud's work, and giving an account of problems of neurosis.

Bruch, H., *Eating Disorders: Obesity, Anorexia Nervosa and the Person Within*, Basic Books Inc. (New York, 1973). An excellent account of the psychological problems met with in obese and anorexic patients.

Burrows, G. D. and Davies, B. (eds), *Handbook of studies on anxiety*, Elsevier (North Holland, 1980). A review of the many aspects of anxiety.

11

PSYCHOTHERAPY AND BEHAVIOUR THERAPY

INTRODUCTION

Psychotherapy is a specialty within psychiatry and refers to a number of specialized methods of psychological treatments (i.e. talking treatments) that can be:

(1) One of the many forms of treatment directed towards cure or amelioration of symptoms, particularly for patients suffering from psychoneuroses, disorders of personality and sexual problems.

(2) A way of promoting psychological development in individuals who have 'hold ups' in their personal developments, which cause problems in *interpersonal relationships* rather than in causing symptoms.

Disturbances of interpersonal relationships are a cardinal feature of many psychiatric problems. Psychiatry itself has even been defined as a study of interpersonal relationships. Such disturbances can be due to specific psychiatric syndromes such as depression, schizophrenia or dementia, e.g. the changes in family relationships produced by a depressed housewife. Many psychiatric patients have longstanding problems in their relationships with other people in the absence of a specific psychiatric syndrome. Dominance, dependence and hostility are perhaps the main problems and show themselves in the family setting and at work.

The traditional individual psychotherapy of one patient and one doctor has been complemented in recent years by settings where one therapist treats groups of people, e.g. conjoint therapy with a married couple; family therapy and group therapy.

In addition psychotherapies can be classified along a continuum from supportive therapy (see chapter 9) at one end to 'uncovering' therapies at the other. With supportive therapies the aim is to support the patient's defences and coping mechanisms. With uncovering therapies the aims are to achieve greater insight, it is these that will be considered in more detail here. It is important to emphasize that such psychotherapy is a specialized technique and should not be attempted by the unskilled without guidance. As has been mentioned supportive care is of value in most patients and it is only a minority of psychiatric patients who need intensive psychotherapy. A doctor who is not a psychiatrist should limit his 'psychotherapy' to interested listening, environmental manipulation, explanations, reassurance, advice, persuasion and re-education. He should *not* uncover dynamic material by free association or dream analysis or give interpretations. Nor should he use hypnosis, or 'abreact' patients with intravenous barbiturates. The reason for this is that complex emotional situations develop during psychotherapy. The feelings which the patient develops towards the therapist often mirror his childhood reactions to his parents, and are regarded as being a *transference* from parents to therapist. The unskilled psychotherapist will not recognize these *transference situations* nor his own emotional reactions to the patient *(counter-transference)*. These complex issues can confound the situation to the patient's detriment and so increase the problems of treatment.

Psychotherapists are usually psychiatrists who have spent several years training in psychotherapy, and this training ensures that these transference problems can be dealt with for the patient's benefit. Patients with a history of grossly disturbed childhood or with sexual problems usually develop these transference problems quickly.

Indications for Psychotherapy

In the last chapter some general remarks were made about the sort of neurotic patient who should be referred for psychotherapy. Other patients who might benefit from psychotherapy are those with some of the personality features described in chapter 6, and with the sexual problems described in chapter 23. Certain alcoholic and drug dependent patients may also benefit from psychotherapy.

Contraindications for Psychotherapy

Most schizophrenic and severely depressed patients are not candidates for psychotherapy, neither are patients with organic brain syndromes.

Methods of Psychotherapy

Patients referred for psychotherapy are usually seen by the therapist on several occasions before a decision is taken to embark on formal treatment. Such treatment then means the patient will be actively involved with the therapist for a 50 minute session, once, twice, or three times a week, for several months. In formal psychoanalysis the patient may be seen five days a week for several years in this way. The methods of psychoanalysis developed by Freud are those of *free association* on the part of the patient and *interpretation* by the analyst of preconscious and unconscious material. The analyst also relies extensively on interpretations of the patient's resistances and of the transference situation. This transference relationship is encouraged by the structure of the analytic interview which is standardized. The patient lies on a couch to promote relaxation, free association and the production of unconscious material. The analyst sits out of the patient's vision in order to minimize the inhibition of free association. The relationship between the analyst and the patient is restricted to the analytic sessions and and any social contact is avoided. Because of expense and availability of analysts' time, this form of treatment can involve only a relatively small number of psychiatric patients.

Psychotherapy of briefer duration but based on psychoanalytic principles is however widely used in the treatment of neurosis. Interviews are usually at weekly intervals for perhaps 3 to 6 months. This form of psychotherapy is more readily available than psychoanalysis. The patient usually does not lie down; free association is not often used. The patient is encouraged to talk freely and in detail about all aspects of his life. Interpretations are used, as is the analysis of dreams. While different therapists use different methods the essential ingredient of the therapy is one in which the patient and therapist actively work together. The doctor is deeply involved with his patient, yet he is detached and able to view the relationship objectively. His acceptance of the patient and his problems is of great importance.

In general, methods of 'brief psychotherapy' concentrate on those areas of the patient's life which are most relevant to the problems he faces and the symptoms his displays. Even with a dozen interviews of 45 minutes' duration, once a week, a skilled psychotherapist can accomplish a good deal. Most of this time will be spent by the patient talking about his symptoms and problems in detail, while the doctor listens, accepts and encourages. It is not what the doctor tells the patient, but what he can encourage the patient to tell him that is important.

Part of the time will be spent in the therapist interpreting the patient's resistances and in trying to make the patient recognize his 'life pattern of behaviour'. In brief psychotherapy the principles of supportive care are also used by the therapist.

Most patients are seen individually in this way, but in group therapy 6–10 patients meet together with the therapist once or twice a week. The problems that present in the group situations are even more complex than in individual therapy. Communications within the group are free and are treated in much the same way as the free association of a patient in analysis. Attention is however often directed more to the functioning of the group, and interactions within the group, rather than to the more personal problems of the individual patient. Group therapy is a method of treatment that is of increasing importance because of the number of patients who need psychotherapy and the limited number of psychotherapists available.

CRISIS THERAPY

In recent years attention has been focused on helping people at times of crisis, e.g. severe illness or bereavement. The word crisis refers to the person's emotional reaction to the hazard and not to the event itself. At these times the individual faces an obstacle to important goals which he cannot overcome by his customary modes of behaviour. There are adaptive and maladaptive ways of dealing with such a crisis. Crises may be the periods for maximal effective intervention. However it is often important to work with the families of individuals in crisis and not the individual alone. Students will meet these problems of crisis in their patients who have made suicide attempts.

HYPNOSIS

Hypnosis is a fascinating subject. Its study at the end of the last century and particularly its relationship to hysteria led to the development of psychopathological theories. Early in his work Freud abandoned hypnosis as a method of treatment as he claimed the results were short-lived. The use of hypnosis in psychiatric treatment has tended to fluctuate, particularly because of the development of physical methods of treatment and psychotherapy—at present there is a world-wide growth of popularity. This has in part resulted from the development of biomodification and biofeedback techniques. Some psychiatrists find it a valuable therapeutic method to use in the course of psychotherapy, in selected patients with neurotic symptoms or personality disorder, e.g. anxiety states, phobic illness, hysterical conversion and dissociative reactions. It has also been mentioned that hypnosis should not be used or attempted by the unskilled. Hypnosis has some value in acute painful situations, e.g. labour and dental extractions, but drugs are easier to administer and are more reliable. It can also be useful in the management of chronic pain.

BEHAVIOUR THERAPY

In recent years there has been an increasing use of a group of techniques called *behaviour therapy or behavioural psychotherapy*. This approach is based on the flexible application of principles derived from psychological theories of learning and conditioning, initially developed in the experimental laboratory.

The theories of operant (or instrumental) conditioning, (which includes reward and avoidance training), and of classical conditioning form the main theoretical framework of behaviour therapy. Behaviour therapy is used for some patients with specific psychiatric signs and symptoms such as anxiety, phobias and obsessive-compulsive symptoms, as well as disordered behaviour patterns, such as enuresis and stuttering.

As with other types of psychotherapy, there is considerable debate concerning the degree to which the actual techniques used, correspond to the theoretical concepts and the extent to which their application are the effective ingredients of treatment.

Most behaviour therapists are clinical psychologists, but the techniques are being increasingly employed by a wide range of health professionals in many treatment and rehabilitation settings.

In this approach the patient's problems are regarded as either:

(1) inappropriate or maladaptive habits, which have been learned (e.g. phobias) and which continue to be maintained by particular environmental stimuli; or

(2) the absence of an essential behavioural function resulting from a failure to learn adaptive responses (e.g. speech production in autistic children).

In the first case the behaviour therapists attempt to modify the experience of the patient by various counter-conditioning techniques, conditioned avoidance procedures or punishment techniques, so as to produce 'unlearning' or extinction or suppression of the unwanted habits. In the second case, various measures such as positive and negative operant reinforcements (which increase the probability (or strength) of emission of a response), are employed to increase the likelihood of the desired response.

With behaviour therapy, while there has recently been increasing concern with *covert* aspects of behaviour, the focus is generally on the patient's *overt* behaviour. It is held that changing the way one *acts* effects changes in thoughts and feelings rather than vice versa, as is the general assumption in some other psychotherapies. It is held, for instance, that the *symptoms are the neurosis* and extinction of the learned habits and conditioned responses which they represent, leads to permanent recovery without any need to attend to 'inner', underlying psychopathology. There is a tendency to ignore whatever symbolic meaning a symptom or behavioural pattern may be held to represent, and instead, to direct attention and treatment solely to the symptom or behavioural pattern. Interpretations of the relationship the patient obtains with the therapist and the development of insight into this are not part of the treatment. Treatment concentrates on the maladaptive habits existing in the present and the conditions that maintain them. The approach is less concerned with the historical development of the symptoms than some of the dynamic psychotherapies.

Many specific techniques have been described. Probably the most common form involves a combination of two separate techniques:

(a) *Desensitization*

This is a method of systematic habituation applied when an appropriate pattern of response (e.g. fear, disgust) has been acquired in relation to a particular object or event. Conditions are arranged to ensure repeated exposure to the stimulus situation, at sufficiently low levels of intensity so that the previous response pattern is not completely evoked. Then after a time it is found that further exposures at gradually increasing levels of intensity no longer elicit the former inappropriate response.

(b) *Reciprocal inhibition*

Here the principle involves arranging conditions so that a more appropriate response (one which is compatible with and antagonistic to that usually elicited) occurs in relation to the troublesome situation. Usually a pattern of relaxation is first learned and then transferred to a situation so that it becomes systematically associated with the stimuli which have previously elicited fear. This relaxation response is incompatible with the previous anxiety, leading to inhibition of the latter.

An example of one form of behaviour therapy can be given. A patient with phobic symptoms, develops anxiety symptoms in some particular situation, e.g. leaving home alone. Inquiry will show that anxiety symptoms also occur in other situations, but to a lesser extent, while in some places the patient is able to feel at ease. A detailed history is first taken and list of hierarchies established. At the top is the situation in which the patient becomes most disturbed, and at the bottom the situation in which the patient feels most completely at ease. The therapist then teaches the patient to relax completely. When this has been accomplished the therapist asks the patient to imagine that she is in the situation at the bottom of the hierarchy list. The patient then imagines each step in the hierarchy, while at the same time the therapist helps the patient to stay relaxed. This gradual 'hierarchical desensitization in imagination' takes several sessions. When the patient is able to stay relaxed while thinking of the most distressing situation, then the patient is moved to the real situation, initially in the presence of the therapist. The process is a gradual one but produces good results particularly when the phobic symptoms are confined to a particular situation, e.g. travel in aeroplanes.

A number of variations can be introduced, e.g. the patient may be helped to relax by use of instruments that show him when his muscles are tense (biofeedback technique). Relaxant drugs and hypnosis can also be used to facilitate relaxation.

Other techniques include:

(1) *Flooding (implosive) therapy*

Here (with his prior consent) the patient is exposed to the feared situation. Although considerable anxiety is usually produced the patient is kept in the situation until there is an extinction of severe anxiety.

(2) *Aversion Therapy*

Here an attempt is made to establish a conditioned aversion to an unwanted habit. An aversive stimulus, e.g. electric shock (pain), or nauseant drug (apomorphine), is either (i) systematically paired with the situational stimulus which elicits the inappropriate or unwanted response, or (ii) applied in association with the situational cues and withdrawn only after the required alternative response has occurred.

These measures have been used in the treatment of various drug addictions, some sexual problems, and are considered by some to be operating in the 'bell and pad' treatment of nocturnal enuresis.

(3) Operant conditioning procedures

Positive reinforcement is provided by applying a positive or rewarding consequence whenever the desired response occurs. Such reinforcement can be delivered according to various prearranged schedules. Negative reinforcement involves exposing the patient to an unpleasant or aversive stimulus beforehand and then immediately removing the stimulus after the response which is sought has occurred.

(4) Modelling (imitation) techniques

These methods are based on the observation that imitation plays an important part in influencing behaviour. In treatment, for instance, a child who has developed a phobic response to a particular situation such as a feared animal, can be shown in real life (or on a film) another person (the model) who does not respond with fear but shows affection for the animal.

(5) Extinction techniques

These treatments apply classical conditioning principles with the aim of progressively weakening unwanted motor habits through repeated withholding of the reinforcements (extinction) which have followed the responses in the past.

The negative practice (or massed practice) techniques used in the management of tics, nailbiting, thumb-sucking, and stuttering is a specific form of application of this principle where the patient is instructed to practise the undesired response deliberately and repeatedly. It is supposed that such repetition of the response produces a negative consequence such as fatigue which, in turn, reduces the likelihood of its occurrence.

Many other specific techniques and variants have been developed and applied for the treatment of specific behavioural disturbances. Recently much attention has been directed towards methods of establishing voluntary control over the cognitive factors influencing autonomic functioning. Modification of behaviour has been found to lead to changes in attitudes and the role of cognitive factors in such procedures as mental rehearsal leading to greater self control is being increasingly appreciated.

The whole field of the behavioural psychotherapies is a growing one, both in regard to practical treatment and research. It is too early to estimate precisely the extent to which they will become part of routine psychiatric practice but its contributions have already been considerable.

Problems in Assessing Psychotherapy and Behaviour Therapy

This is an extremely difficult but important question that cannot be completely answered. Adequately controlled trials of the effectiveness of these treatments have not been achieved. Among the many factors difficult to control are the tendency for neurotic symptoms to improve spontaneously over the course of 1–3 years. Patients and therapists differ considerably, as do the techniques used. Nor is neurosis a single disease entity like appendicitis.

Further the *quality of improvement* with these therapies cannot be assessed merely by recording changes in symptoms; a true measure of change is difficult.

However, while the value of these treatments is a subject for debate and investigations, students should recognize that referral of a patient to an experienced general psychiatrist should be the first step in decision making about the need for psychotherapy or behaviour therapy.

Features Common to the Psychotherapies and Behaviour Therapy

Recent studies have drawn attention to the common features of many forms of treatment in psychiatry that include psychotherapy, behaviour therapy, hypnosis and the 'non-pharmacological' response to drug treatments.

In studying different forms of psychotherapy, J. D. Frank has suggested that all psychotherapies have the following common features: (they are also common to all types of 'healers' in all societies and times).

(1) There is an intense, emotionally charged, confiding relationship with a helping person, often with the participation of a group.

(2) There is a rationale, or myth, which includes an explanation of the cause of the patient's distress and a method of relieving it. To be effective, the therapeutic myth must be compatible with the culture of both therapist and patient.

(3) Provision of new information concerning the nature and sources of the patient's problems and possible ways of dealing with them.

(4) Strengthening the patient's expectations of help through the personal qualities of the therapist, enhanced by his status in society and the setting in which he works.

(5) Provision of success experiences which further heighten the patient's hopes and also enhance his sense of mastery and interpersonal competence.

(6) The facilitation of emotional arousal seems to be a prerequisite to attitudinal and behavioural changes.

SUMMARY

Psychotherapy and behaviour therapy are specialized areas of psychiatry. An outline is given of the principles of these forms of treatment; attention is drawn to the common features of these methods of treatment.

REFERENCES

PSYCHOTHERAPY

Bloch, S., *An Introduction to the Psychotherapies,* Oxford Medical Publications (1979). A very useful overview of the whole field of psychotherapy.

Kubie, L. S., *Practical and Theoretical Aspects of Psychoanalysis,* International Universities Press (New York, 1974). This book provides a good understanding of the psychoanalytic viewpoint.

Meares, R. A., *The Shaping Fantasies—an approach to psychotherapy,* Hogarth (London, 1976). Written as an introduction for psychotherapists.

Yalom, I., *Theory and Practice of Group Psychotherapy,* 2nd edn, Basic Books (New York, 1975). Discusses the practical and theoretical aspects of group psychotherapy.

BEHAVIOUR THERAPY

Beech, H. R., *Changing Man's Behaviour,* Penguin Books (Harmondsworth, 1969).

Meyer, V. and Chesser, E. S., *Behaviour Therapy in Clinical Psychiatry,* Penguin Books (Harmondsworth, 1970).

Yates, Aubrey J., *Behaviour Therapy,* John Wiley & Sons (New York, 1970).

GENERAL PAPERS

Frank, J. D., 'Common features of psychotherapy', *Australia and New Zealand Journal of Psychiatry,* vol. 6 (1972), p. 34.

Marks, I., 'The future of the psychotherapies', *British Journal of Psychiatry,* no. 118 (1971), pp. 69–73.

Sloane, R. B., 'The converging paths of behaviour therapy and psychotherapy', *American Journal of Psychiatry,* no. 125 (1969), pp. 877–85.

12

DEPRESSIVE ILLNESS AND ITS TREATMENT

Perhaps the most important task for students in their study of psychiatry is to learn how to recognize and treat mild to moderately severe depressive illness. There are several reasons for this:

(1) It is a common illness that is often associated with physical illness.
(2) Many of the symptoms of depressive illness can suggest physical illness, and many fruitless investigations of the patient can be made if the depression is not recognized.
(3) Suicide is an important complication of depressive illness.
(4) Depressive illness is now an eminently treatable condition.

DEFINITION

Depressive illness is an illness of mood, i.e., an affective disorder. The actual neurophysiological basis of mood control is not clearly defined, yet most people experience a fairly constant mood, with only brief changes, either elevation or lowering of mood. In affective disorders there is a *fixed change of mood* which profoundly influences behaviour and thinking. In depressive illness there is a persistent lowering of mood, while in the uncommon manic illness there is a persistent elevation of mood.

CLINICAL FEATURES

There are a number of symptoms that are associated with this lowered mood and they are called *depressive symptoms*.

DEPRESSIVE SYMPTOMS

(1) *Mood Change*
This is present in all depressed patients, and is the essential abnormality. There is a feeling of sadness that can range from mild despondency to abject despair that overwhelms the patient. Every patient is aware of this change in his or her feeling state, yet few complain spontaneously of it, particularly in the early stages of the illness. There is a great variation in how patients describe this mood change. Patients must be asked, 'Have you been feeling miserable lately?—Have you felt like crying?—How do you feel in yourself?'

(2) *Loss of Interest*
Perhaps the next most important symptom is the loss of interest that accompanies the lowered mood. Patients again will not usually

mention this. Loss of interest in the house, work, hobbies, recreation and religion are most important symptoms of depressive illness, as is loss of sexual interest. Loss of interest in personal appearance and hygiene is a most significant sign.

(3) *Sleep Disturbance*

This is often the earliest symptom of a depressive illness. Sometimes however, it is overlooked as the patient has been given sleeping tablets and forgets to mention that he had never needed hypnotics until a few months previously. Patients may complain that they cannot get to sleep because of their worries and when they sleep they have disturbing dreams. Other patients may say they fall asleep quite easily but wake up early in the morning, cannot sleep again, and feel particularly depressed.

(4) *Difficulty in Thinking and Concentrating*

Patients with depressive illness cannot concentrate on simple tasks like reading or housework. They find it difficult to converse or to make decisions. Elderly patients with depression may do badly on tests of memory because of these difficulties and a wrong diagnosis of dementia may be made (chapter 16).

(5) *Painful Thoughts*

The depressed patient becomes preoccupied with himself; his thoughts are painful and concerned with his liabilities. He cannot 'count his blessings'. He blames himself, magnifies his misdeeds and worries over any minor problems. He ruminates over the past and his peccadilloes. The present and future appear black.

(6) *Suicidal Thoughts*

Depressed patients, because of the mood change and these painful thoughts, often have suicidal thoughts. They should be asked about these. 'Have you thought that life is not worth living?' Most depressed patients will recognize these thoughts and are helped by being asked to talk about them.

(7) *Anxiety*

Depressed patients are usually anxious. It is important not to miss depressive symptoms in some patients who present with anxiety. Anxious depressed patients are often restless and this motor restlessness is called *agitation*. It varies in degree from mild to severe.

(8) *Hypochondriasis*

Anxious concern over general health or conviction of a particular disease is a most important symptom of depressive illness.

(9) *Irritability*

Undue or unusual irritability, particularly at home, is an important depressive symptom.

(10) *Paranoid Ideas*

Depressed patients often think that people are against them and know about their defects. These ideas are in keeping with the depressed mood.

(11) *Retardation*

Depressed patients become slow in their movements and in severe cases the patient can become stuporous. By contrast their thinking often seems to be speeded up—particularly with circular worrying thoughts about the past or future.

Physical Complaints in Depressive Illness

Nearly half the patients with depressive illness first report to the doctor with complaints that suggest physical illness. If the above depressive symptoms are not enquired about, the diagnosis of depression may be overlooked and many fruitless investigations made. Such complaints are:

(1) Fatigue and tiredness
(2) Anorexia and consequent weight loss
(3) Constipation
(4) Menstrual changes
(5) Bodily aches and pains
(6) Headaches
(7) Difficulty in breathing
(8) Dryness of the mouth
(9) Unusual sensations in the abdomen, chest or head may be *interpreted by the doctor* as dyspepsia, dyspnoea or headaches. If the *actual phenomenology* is enquired into, these errors will not occur

These 'physical' symptoms are caused by changes in bodily functions associated with the depressive illness, mediated through the autonomic nervous system.

SIGNS

The facial appearance of most depressed patients is characteristic with a furrowed brow, immobile face, down-turned mouth and an expression of troubled perplexity. Students should learn to recognize this at a glance. The stooped posture and slowed movements, or the restless agitation are also important signs.

It is the persistence of these depressive symptoms and signs that make up the syndrome of depressive illness. It is important to recognize that clinically:

(1) Depressive symptoms occur in many physical and psychiatric illnesses. They form a subsidiary part of the symptomatology and are often a reaction to the main illness. This association, as will be mentioned, is of the greatest importance in general medical practice (see chapter 13). Any acute or chronic medical condition may be associated with depressive symptoms. Psychiatric illnesses frequently associated with depression, are chronic brain syndromes and schizophrenia.

68

The patient's prognosis in these cases is dependent upon that of the main condition, though the depressive symptoms may be relieved with treatment.

(2) *In primary depressive illness,* the predominant feature is the persistent mood change from which the depressive symptoms and signs stem.

ONSET AND COURSE

The onset is usually gradual over the course of a few months, but can be abrupt, and a florid illness may develop in a few days.

The course of the illness is a self-limiting one. Before the days of active treatment it was known that illnesses of mood (depression or mania) remitted completely, leaving the patient as he was before the illness came on. It was also known that some patients tended to get further attacks of depression or mania.

The actual length of the illness is very variable. The mild form (particularly in the elderly) tends to be more chronic than the severe which often develops acutely. In general, without treatment most severe depressive illnesses would have cleared within a year, and it would be unusual for symptoms to persist for more than 2 years.

CULTURAL AND SOCIAL FACTORS, AGE AND SEX

Depressive illness occurs throughout the world but is probably more frequent in people of European origin.

It is evenly distributed throughout the social classes in Britain and the United States.

Depressive illness occurs at all ages from childhood to advanced age, but is more frequent in the 50s, 60s and 70s. This also corresponds to the peak age for suicide. Women are more liable to depressive symptoms than men.

PRECIPITATING FACTORS

Certain events are not infrequently followed by depressive symptoms:

(1) Physical illness or operations; particularly in the elderly. (Influenza and infective hepatitis are two common illnesses that can be followed by depressive symptoms.)

(2) Bereavement (see chapter 13).

(3) Pregnancy and parturition (see chapter 22).

(4) Certain drugs—reserpine, Aldomet and the contraceptive pill—may be factors in producing depression.

TYPES OF DEPRESSIVE ILLNESS

There is a wide range of severity of depressive illness and the question arises whether the term 'depressive illness' covers a number of different syndromes? In the absence of a demonstrable pathology or of specific physiological disturbances such a question can only be answered clinically.

In clinical practice there seem to be two *contrasting* types of depressive illness, and a third which has elements of both types.

Endogenous Depression

In the predominantly *endogenous* type of depression, symptoms are thought to be determined to a large extent by genetic-constitutional factors. The symptoms are usually severe, and the onset may have been independent of adverse environmental circumstances (though precipitation by the factors already mentioned is common). Symptoms tend to be worse in the morning and improve later in the day (diurnal variation), while the patient tends to wake early in the morning. Loss of weight and sex drive may be marked. Perhaps most characteristic is the fact that the depressed mood is not altered by pleasing environmental circumstances.

Reactive Depression

In the predominantly *reactive* type of depression, symptoms are understandable as a reaction of a particular sort of personality to a particular situation. Often the situation is one which has produced anger or hostility in the patient and depressive symptoms follow. Symptoms are usually variable and mild and tend to be worse in the evening. Anxiety symptoms are usually prominent. Patients find it difficult to fall off to sleep because of worrying thoughts about the events of the day. The symptoms respond (albeit temporarily) to favourable environmental circumstances. This syndrome with anxiety and depression is the most frequently diagnosed neurotic group of symptoms (see chapter 10). Patients with reactive depression are usually younger than those with the endogenous type.

Mixed Depression

There is a *mixed* type in which features of both endogenous and reactive depression are present.

Statistical evaluation of clinical data, using methods of factor analysis, has given support to the clinical distinction between reactive and endogenous depression. There is as yet no physiological or biochemical way of distinguishing these types of depressive illness; or indeed any such tests that can distinguish a depressed person from someone with a normal mood.

Psychiatrists in psychiatric hospitals will see mainly endogenous depression, general practitioners mainly reactive depressions, while in outpatient and general hospital work mixed pictures are usual.

What matters in each patient is the recognition of the symptoms present and their severity as judged by the way they have interfered with the patient's life and the assessment of possible causative factors. Some illnesses clearly fall into the 'endogenous' group, and some into the 'reactive' group; but many do not and it is *not important* in these last cases to decide 'endogenous' or 'reactive'.

Modern techniques of cluster analysis of depressive phenomenology have suggested four types of depression:

(1) A severe depression in older patients often with delusions and a good premorbid personality.

There are usually no precipitating events (i.e. 'endogenous').

(2) A moderately severe depression with high levels of anxiety in middle-aged patients, often with an obsessional personality.

(3) A middle-aged depressed patient with marked hostility and self pitying features in the behaviour and mental state.

(4) A young, anxious group with evidence of precipitating life events, (i.e. 'neurotic or reactive').

HISTORY FROM RELATIVES

A history from the nearest relative is of great importance in diagnosing depressive illness. The student should recognize that *he* cannot compare the patient's present state with his usual self. Only someone who has known the patient for some time can do this. Some patients who do not appear severely depressed have been active energetic people prior to their illness, and the illness may even seem to 'normalize' them. Yet in fact this sort of depressive illness can have the same suicidal risk as more obviously depressed patients.

RELATIONSHIP OF MANIA TO DEPRESSION

It has been noted in historical medical writings that there is an occasional association of manic and depressive attacks in the same patient (bipolar). This is unusual. Depressive illness alone (unipolar) is commonest. Manic illness alone is an uncommon illness that is essentially the concern of the psychiatrist. The symptoms are the exact converse of depression—elation—grandiose thoughts—overactivity and pressure of talk and activity. Sleep is disturbed and sex drive increased.

HYPOCHONDRIASIS

Hypochondriacal symptoms are frequent in depressive illness, but usually the cardinal symptoms and signs of a depressive illness are also present. Some patients are seen who have had marked hypochondriacal symptoms for many years, yet lack the other definite symptoms of depressive illness. It is often best to treat these patients with antidepressive medication, as some of them respond satisfactorily.

FUNDAMENTAL CAUSES OF DEPRESSIVE ILLNESS

It has been mentioned already that depressive illness is an illness of mood, and that its actual neurophysiological basis is not yet known. In recent years much research interest has centred about the chemical basis of mood. Clinical observations on the actions of three drugs, reserpine, iproniazid and imipramine led to suggestions about the biochemical basis of disorders of mood. Studies have suggested changes in brain monoamines (the catecholamines and indoleamines) are related to *severe* disorders of mood. A monoamine hypothesis could be stated thus 'that depressive illnesses are associated with a relative deficiency of certain monoamines in certain parts of the brain. Antidepressant treatments produce improvement by altering monoamine metabolism in certain parts of the brain. The converse applies to mania and anti-manic treatments.'

It has been shown by studies of twins and families of depressed patients that there is a *genetic* predisposition to depressive illness, though this may not become manifest till late in life and in the presence of precipitating factors, e.g., bereavement or a cerebrovascular accident.

Psychopathological theories that stem from Freud's study *On Mourning and Melancholia* have given important insights into psychological mechanisms of depression. In particular the *loss* of some source of self esteem can, in some people with a certain personality structure, cause depression. This loss may be bereavement, or physical health, loss of status on retiring, loss of home, property, etc. These factors may be important in some patients with depressive illness, but are by no means always present.

DIFFERENTIAL DIAGNOSIS

Physical Causes

The many symptoms that depressed patients may complain of can suggest the presence of many diseases. In excluding *physical causes*, a full physical examination and if necessary, ancillary investigations may be needed. Frequent clinical problems are neoplasms, anaemia and myxoedema.

The *common association* of depressive symptoms and physical disease will be mentioned in chapter 16.

Anxiety

Patients who present with anxiety symptoms often have a depressive illness and enquiry into all depressive symptoms is important. Other anxious patients do not have depressive symptoms (see chapter 10). It is important to try and decide about this because treatment with anti-depressive or anti-anxiety drugs may be an essential part of the management of the patient. These will be discussed later.

Hysteria

Hysterical illness *per se* is uncommon, though hysterical symptoms are frequent and can be precipitated by a depressive illness. Here again enquiry into all depressive symptoms is important. Again it is important to decide whether to treat the hysterical symptoms with anti-depressive treatment or by other means.

Obsessional Symptoms

Obsessional symptoms are frequent in depressive illness. These symptoms occurring for the first time in an elderly patient are due to the presence of a depressive illness. In all patients with obsessional symptoms an important practical question is whether to use anti-depressive treatment or tranquillizing drugs in the total management of the patient.

Neurotic Personality

It is apparent in clinical work that many patients with a history of long standing neurotic personality features may present with an exacerbation of these symptoms, be they anxiety, phobic, obsessional or hysterical ones. This exacerbation often is due to the development of a depressive illness though the depressive symptoms can be overlooked by the inexperienced. *These patients are important, as the appropriate treatment may be supportive care and anti-depressive treatment and not psychotherapy.*

Schizophrenia

In depression (and mania) thought content is appropriate to the mood disorder. This may not be so in schizophrenia. Complex paranoid ideas are more usually due to schizophrenia.

TREATMENT

Once depressive symptoms are recognized, the next question is whether they are associated with another well-defined illness (physical or psychiatric) or not.

The next problem for the general practitioner is whether to treat the patient himself or refer him to a psychiatrist.

Patients with severe symptoms and suicidal ideas are best admitted to hospital under psychiatric care. The following features are usually regarded as indicating a significant risk of suicide in depressed patients:

(1) Suicidal preoccupations
(2) Marked guilt feelings and self-depreciation.
(3) Agitation
(4) Severe hypochondriasis
(5) Sleeplessness and concern over it
(6) A history of a previous depressive illness with a suicide attempt
(7) Being alone, or an unsympathetic attitude of the family (this is particularly so in elderly patients who live alone)
(8) Presence of serious physical illness
(9) Alcohol or drug addiction
(10) Financial difficulties
(11) Depression in patients with a history of a severely deprived childhood.

73

Electro-Convulsive Therapy (E.C.T.)

The most effective treatment for *these severely depressed patients* is a course of electro-convulsive therapy. Its actual mode of action is unknown, but there is no more dramatic sight in medicine than to see a severely agitated melancholic revert to normal in the course of 3-4 weeks. Treatments are usually given two or three times a week, with intravenous barbiturates and muscle relaxants, so that the muscular effects of the fit are completely modified. The procedure is safe, and the only contra-indications are a recent myocardial or cerebrovascular accident. Most depressed patients need between 6-12 treatments before improvement is complete.

Students should be aware of the value of E.C.T. in severe depression but should be fully informed about the treatment of the moderate and mild illnesses that they will meet in the general hospital and in general practice.

THE DRUG TREATMENT OF DEPRESSION
The Tricyclic Group of Anti-depressant Drugs

These compounds which are *iminodibenzyl* derivatives, differ chemically from the M.A.O.I. drugs, and because of their less serious side effects are now *the anti-depressants of first choice. Imipramine* (Tofranil) was the first of these compounds; it has a chemical structure similar to that of chlorpromazine, and was first used in 1957. These drugs, like the M.A.O.I., alter the metabolism of brain monoamines (but by a different mechanism). In addition, these drugs may act via their anti-cholinergic effect at the synaptic or neuronal level, modifying cholinergic activity which seems to be related to some depressive states. Imipramine is not an M.A.O.I. or a cerebral stimulant. Dosage is usually 150 mg per day. Improvement may not occur until tablets have been taken for 3-6 weeks at full dosage. Side effects (*of which patients should be warned*) include dryness of the mouth, constipation, sweating and disturbances in accommodation. Tremors and a mild parkinsonian syndrome can develop. In addition, orthostatic hypotension and urinary retention (in men) can be problems, while epilepsy can be provoked.

Another drug related to imipramine is amitryptyline (Tryptanol, Elavil, Laroxyl). This drug has similar anti-depressant properties but is more sedative and may be more useful in agitated depressed patients.

Because these drugs do not cause vascular or liver damage they are the most valuable drugs at present available in the treatment of depressive illness. Suicidal attempts with these drugs are dangerous because of cardiac arrhythmias.

The Monoamine Oxidase Inhibitors

The treatment of depressive illness has completely altered since the introduction of the first anti-depressant drug iproniazid (Marsilid) in

74

1956. This was used to treat chronic tuberculosis, but it was noticed that some of the patients became euphoric and actual mania was observed. Following these observations the drug was used in 1956 in depressed patients and, in a number of trials, recovery rates ranged from 30% to 70%. Iproniazid inhibits the action of the enzyme monoamine oxidase which occurs widely in the body. In the C.N.S. these monoamine oxidase inhibitors (M.A.O.I.) increase the levels of the various monoamines, and it has been suggested that these changes may underlie the value of these drugs in depressive illness. (Note that *reserpine*, used to treat hypertension, lowers the levels of brain serotonin and catecholamines and severe depression is a well known side effect of reserpine treatment.)

The usual daily dose of iproniazid is 75-100 mg. Side effects reported with iproniazid include hypertension, hypomania, oedema, impotence and most important, fatal liver necrosis. *Because of this last side effect, the use of this drug is now limited.*

Other M.A.O.I. have been developed that are *relatively* free from toxic effects on the liver. Daily dosage should be given before midday to help reduce sleeplessness.

>Phenelzine (Nardil)   —dosage 30-90 mg./day
>Tranylcypromine (Parnate)—dosage 20-50 mg./day
>Isocarboxazid (Marplan)   —dosage 20-60 mg./day

Side Effects of M.A.O.I.

All these drugs can produce side effects which are not uncommon—postural hypotension, nausea, oedema, impotence, sleeplessness. Liver damage is rare with these newer drugs.

Three symptom complexes have been described as complications of treatment with M.A.O.I. They have as a common basis a rapid elevation of systemic blood pressure.

(1) Paroxymal headaches of great intensity (associated with marked elevation of blood pressure). There may also be pallor, chills, neck stiffness and collapse. These symptoms are similar to those that occur in subarachnoid haemorrhage.

(2) Cardiovascular manifestations may be prominent—palpitations, chest pain, hypotension, sweating, pallor, headaches and collapse. These symptoms are similar to those seen with a phaeochromocytoma.

(3) Intracranial haemorrhage

Symptoms are as (1) above, but focal neurological signs or convulsions are found. Diagnosis depends upon finding blood stained cerebrospinal fluid. Patients may make a complete recovery from this incident, or be left with permanent neurological damage, while deaths have occurred.

These side effects were first reported with tranylcypromine (Parnate) but can occur with any M.A.O.I. The attacks are usually precipitated by eating substances containing pressor amines (particularly tyramine).

The M.A.O.I. inhibit the monoamine oxidase in the intestinal wall that normally breaks down these substances. Patients on M.A.O.I. should not eat cheese, Vegemite, creams or alcohol. With dietary restrictions these reactions can be minimized.

The most dangerous side effects of M.A.O.I. are due to their reactions with other drugs. It is more difficult to prevent these. Severe and fatal reactions with hyperpyrexia, nausea, vomiting and collapse have been reported in patients who are taking M.A.O.I. and who have been given amphetamines (including nasal decongestants), adrenaline, ephedrine, diuretics, anti-parkinsonian drugs, morphia, pethidine, steroids, tranquillizers, local and general anaesthetics and the imipramine group of drugs (see later). Bee stings have caused death.

Another distinct drawback of the M.A.O.I. drugs is that if they are ineffective in depressive illness, at least two weeks must elapse after stopping them before other anti-depressant drugs can be used. It takes time for the body to eliminate M.A.O.I. and the severe reactions with the other drugs mentioned above can occur during this withdrawal period.

There can be no doubt that M.A.O.I. are valuable in some patients with depression, yet the side effects mentioned above make their use a real problem for the family doctor.

The Value of Anti-depressant Drugs

Many of the reports on the value of these anti-depressant drugs are uncontrolled and valid conclusions cannot be made from them.

Clinical improvement occurring during the course of drug administration is not necessarily due to the pharmacological properties of the drug. This dictum is particularly important with depressive illness, the course of which can be influenced significantly by many factors within the patient and his environment.

Many of the conflicting reports about the value of these drugs depend upon the wide range in the severity of depressive illness and the fluctuations in the symptoms that are part of the natural history of the illness. These drugs have, however, stimulated a great deal of research into the neurophysiological and biochemical basis of mood and mood deviation.

New Anti-depressant Drugs

In recent years some new anti-depressants have been introduced. They have fewer unpleasant side effects (e.g. dry mouth, constipation, urinary retention) than the currently used tricyclic compounds, and they have little or no cardiotoxic side effect and are therefore relatively safe on overdosage. These drugs are now widely used as the anti-depressants of first choice in the elderly and in depressed patients with heart disease. However, their clinical efficacy as anti-depressants requires more study. Such drugs include: mianserin

(Tolvon), 10 mg. tablets, daily dosage 40-80 mg.; maprotiline (Ludiomil), 25 mg. tablets, daily dosage 75-300 mg. Nomifensine and zimelidine are two other such compounds.

These, and other compounds, all have different chemical structures and pharmacological actions from the standard anti-depressants. This has given rise to new theories of anti-depressant action.

TREATMENT OF DEPRESSION

For *mild* depressive symptoms, treatment is mainly along psychological, social and symptomatic lines (i.e., non-barbiturate hypnotics for sleep disturbance).

For *severe* depressive illness, e.g., patients admitted to psychiatric hospitals, electro-convulsive therapy (E.C.T.) remains the treatment of choice. E.C.T., despite much research and speculation, is an empirical procedure with a negligible mortality rate and with few physical contra-indications. At the present time there is no drug that can match the efficacy of E.C.T. in severe depressive illness in short term results.

For the *moderately severe* depressive illness, the tricyclic anti-depressants are of great value and have completely transformed psychiatric outpatient work. Imipramine (Tofranil) or amitriptyline (Laroxyl, Tryptanol) are the drugs most used. *There is some evidence that daily dosage of these drugs below 150 mg. is no better than placebo.* It has been mentioned that full anti-depressant effects may take several weeks.

More effective and less toxic compounds are being searched for. Their discovery would be of great significance, as present day drugs are not ideal.

TREATMENT WITH ANTIDEPRESSANTS

Introduction

In general practice most patients treated with antidepressants improve, often improving in the first week of treatment.

Such improvement is not due to the antidepressant action of the compound. It is due to the most important ingredients of medical treatment, *the doctor's faith in his treatment and the patient's faith in his doctor.*

This transactional interpersonal relationship is the basis of all good medicine and should not be dismissed as the 'placebo reaction'.

In a controlled trial in some general practices in Melbourne, 75 mg. and 150 mg. of amitriptyline, 150 mg. of amylobarbitone and inert capsules were given to depressed patients each day for 4 weeks. *More than 60 per cent of the patients improved, irrespective of the content of the capsules and most improved in the first week of treatment.* However, 150 mg. of amitriptyline was significantly better than other treatments in relieving anxiety and depressive symptoms over a 4 week period.

The patients who stopped the capsules because of complaints of side effects were equally distributed among the 4 treatment groups (including the inert capsules).

Practical Therapeutics in Depression

(1) The doctor should begin antidepressant treatment with a tricyclic antidepressant either imipramine or amitriptyline or his own favourite tricyclic antidepressant. Initial dosage of imipramine or amitryptyline is 50 mg. at night and 25 mg. in the morning. Patients should be told to expect side effects—dry mouth, constipation and sleepiness. They should be told that these symptoms mean the pills are beginning to work but that the depression won't really begin to improve for 7–14 days.

(2) *The patient should be seen again in 7 days.*

(a) If improvement has already begun and the patient seems well, the medication at the above dose should be continued for a month.

(b) If the patient is still depressed, increase the night dose to 100 mg. and continue the 25 mg. in the morning.

(3) *The patient should be seen again in 7 days.*
If the patient is still unwell increase the dose to 150 mg. per day. 100 mg. at night and 50 mg. in the morning.

(4) *The patient should be seen weekly until improvement is definite. Patients should be given a definite appointment and not told 'come and see me if you are no better'.*
At the end of the 4 weeks most patients will have improved. For those who have not, dosage should be continued at 150–250 mg/day for at least another 3 weeks. *Clinically, patients who are not experiencing side effects are not having a therapeutic dose of drug (they may not even be taking the drug!). If there is no improvement in this time, patients should be referred to a psychiatrist.*

No other drugs should be given with tricyclic drugs if at all possible.

Giving the tricyclic at night usually helps insomnia without adding an hypnotic. If an hypnotic is still needed *never use barbiturates.* They affect the metabolism of tricyclics by increasing liver enzyme activity. If needed diazepam or nitrazepam can be given as hypnotics.

PRACTICAL THERAPEUTIC NOTES

(1) If one tricyclic does not help there is no point in changing to another compound, their metabolites are very similar. It is better to increase the dose of the original compound.

(2) Warnings about alcohol and tricyclics and driving should be given to patients. Patients who have to drive a lot should take all the daily

dose at night and none in the day before driving, (unless they are driving at night in which case the drug should be taken in the morning).

(3) The pharmaceutical companies warn doctors not to prescribe tricyclics (or any drugs) in the first trimester of pregnancy. However, if the clinical condition merits tricyclics, there is no hard evidence that they cause foetal abnormalities.

(4) Tricyclics should be continued for some months after moderately depressed patients improve. As a general rule they should be continued for as long as the symptoms had been present before treatment began, before attempting to reduce the dosage. This should be done gradually, one tablet a week to see if a recurrence occurs. If it does the original dosage should be re-instituted.

Generally in general practice drugs need to be continued for about 3 months. In some patients with longer standing symptoms 6 months is needed. Some patients, treated usually by psychiatrists, need to be taking tricyclics for longer than a year.

(5) There is some evidence that at therapeutic dosage, imipramine and amitriptyline can cause cardiac arrhythmias in patients with heart disease. Preliminary studies suggest that doxepin and mianserin are less likely to do this, so that these are at present recommended for patients with heart disease and depression.

(6) Patients with glaucoma and depression can be treated with tricyclics but need referral to a psychiatrist and ophthalmologist.

(7) Patients with urinary retention also need referral since tricyclics can aggravate this problem though mianserin may not.

(8) Elderly patients with depression usually need energetic treatment with tricyclics. Therapeutic dosage is the same namely 150 mg./day and while attaining this daily dose may take longer, it should be done. *In this respect the 10 mg. tablets often used in the elderly are pharmacologically useless as antidepressants.*

(9) Mixed preparations of an antidepressant and a tranquillizer are available and are widely prescribed. There are some pharmacological grounds for their use, since the phenothiazine tranquillizer increases the amount of tricyclic in the plasma and is an anti anxiety agent. However, the effective antidepressant dose is still 150 mg./day of the amitriptyline contained in these capsules.

(10) Menopausal women are often depressed and respond well to antidepressants. In the long term however, more than this is usually needed. Often some part time activity outside the home is most helpful.

(11) Occasionally starting tricyclic medication can produce an epileptic fit. Usually if the dosage is reduced then increased gradually, drug treatment can still continue. Depressed epileptics who are receiving barbiturates or barbiturate derivatives as treatment for their epilepsy

should be referred for specialist advice, since, as has been mentioned, barbiturates interfere with tricyclic metabolism.

(12) Some patients who are being treated with hypotensive drugs also need treatment with antidepressants. Despite occasional problems of blood pressure control, the drugs can be used together, but again the general practitioner may wish to seek specialist advice. Reserpine and alpha methyl dopa are hypotensive drugs that can actually cause depression.

(13) Depressed patients with severe liver or kidney disease should be referred for specialist advice about antidepressant treatment.

MONOAMINE OXIDASE INHIBITORS

These substances are not the first line of treatment in depression. Their place in practical therapeutics is still debated. *Treatment with these drugs is probably better started by a psychiatrist than a general practitioner.* Among psychiatrists there are enthusiastic and cynical reports about these drugs. They are almost certainly under used bceause of fears about toxic reactions. G.P.s should read the drug information carefully before using them. They are used most often in:

(1) Anxious patients who have severe phobic symptoms as well as depressive symptoms.

(2) In some depressed patients who have responded to them previously.

(3) In some depressed patients who have not responded to tricyclics.

Except for causing difficulty in sleeping, the M.A.O.I. do not produce the unpleasant side effects that tricyclics do. Marplan, Nardil and Parnate do not cause liver damage and are the drugs of choice. All patients treated with these drugs should be given a card (available from the drug companies) that reads:

'*A Word of Caution*'

Your physician has prescribed an effective modern drug for the treatment of your condition. Be sure to follow his directions carefully. Here are a few things to keep in mind while you are taking this medication.

(1) Don't take any other medicines (including cold remedies) without asking your physician.

(2) Don't eat cheese (particularly strong or aged varieties), raisins, chocolate, sour cream, pickled herring, chicken livers, canned figs, avocado pears, the pods of broad beans or protein extracts (Marmite, Vegemite, Bonox, etc.). In general, avoid foods in which ageing is used to increase flavour.

(3) Don't drink alcoholic beverages.

(4) If you are to receive an anaesthetic for surgical or other purposes, advise the physician or dentist in charge that you are taking this drug.

(5) Report promptly to your physician any unusual headache or other symptoms.

(6) If you become pregnant or are likely to do so, discuss with your doctor any drugs you are taking.

SUPPORTIVE CARE

While anti-depressant treatment is most important the principles of supportive care previously described must be applied. *In general practice, where patients with mild and variable depressive symptoms are the rule, supportive care is usually more important than anti-depressant medication.* Depressed patients will need medical care for several months or even several years.

LITHIUM

Cade, in 1948, showed that lithium has a definite effect in relieving the severe psychiatric disturbance seen in manic patients. However the discovery of chlorpromazine in 1952 led to a neglect of research on lithium. In the past 10 years it has become clear that lithium has an important place in preventing recurring attacks of depression and (or) mania.

Lithium is used in patients who have had one hospital admission with an affective illness, for each of two successive years or twice in one year. The drug has to be given daily and the dosage monitored by plasma lithium estimations. The optimal level is about 0.6 m.eq/litre. Some 80 per cent of such patients are significantly helped by this mode of treatment. Such long term treatment has some important side effects that include tremor and effects on the thyroid and kidney. It is best organized from a special lithium clinic.

PSYCHOTHERAPY

Many patients with reactive depression need psychotherapy either in association with drug treatment, or as the only treatment. Suggestions about the sort of patients to refer have been mentioned in chapter 10.

MODIFIED LEUCOTOMY

This operation has a place in the treatment of the uncommon elderly depressed patient whose symptoms do not respond completely to all other forms of treatment. Such symptoms will have been present at least 2 years before the operation is considered. In present day practice, leucotomy is rarely indicated.

SUMMARY

Depressive illness is a persistent disorder of mood; it is a frequent, socially important, treatable illness.

Depressive symptoms are protean; they include many somatic symptoms.

The syndromes of reactive and endogenous depression are defined and methods of assessing suicidal risk are detailed. Treatment with drugs is now an important aspect of the general management of depressive illness.

The anti-depressant drugs are described; they include a tricyclic group and a group of monoamine oxidase inhibitors. It is important to know how to use these drugs properly and to know their side effects (particularly of the M.A.O.I.).

Effective antidepressant medication causes an improvement in outcome of from 55 per cent with inert medication to 75 per cent. This is important clinically. However, the basic 'understanding' aspects of the doctor/patient interaction should not be forgotten in a chemical assault on the patient.

REFERENCE

Burrows, G. (ed.), *Handbook of Studies on Depression*. Excerpta Medica. Elsevier (North Holland, 1980). A review of all aspects of affective disorders.

13

COMBINED PHYSICAL AND PSYCHIATRIC ILLNESS PAIN—EPILEPSY—THE DYING PATIENT— GRIEF AND MOURNING

In general we tend to think of mind and body as separate entities and present medical training fosters a distinction between physical and psychiatric illness. Although there are theoretical objections to this 'dualistic' way of thinking, a distinction between physical and psychological is useful in clinical practice, provided that interactions between body and mind are acknowledged. Throughout these notes emphasis has been placed *on a total approach to the patient as a person, with physical, psychological and social dimensions.* This chapter deals with a number of clinical problems in medicine where this total approach is helpful.

PHYSICAL AND PSYCHIATRIC ILLNESS

Investigations of hospital inpatients and outpatients and in general practice have shown that the combination of physical and psychiatric illness is common, being found in between 20% and 50% of all patients seen.
The usual clinical problems are:
(1) The commonest and most important are patients with chronic physical illness who also have *depressive* or *neurotic* symptoms.
(2) Patients who develop anxiety symptoms in association with an acute physical illness.
(3) Patients who develop an acute brain syndrome (see chapter 15) postoperatively or during the course of a physical illness.
(4) There are still other patients, e.g., chronic alcoholics, and epileptics in whom the physical, psychiatric and social problems are closely interrelated.

History Taking and Physical Examination

Students learn how to take a medical or surgical history in the medical or surgical wards and at the same time learn the methods of physical examination. During their period of psychiatric clerking, students learn to take a psychiatric history and to assess the significance of psychiatric symptoms. At this time the importance of seeing the patient's relatives and trying to picture the patient at home and at work is emphasized.
It is common to have to remind students in the psychiatric wards

that a medical history and a full physical examination is essential for every psychiatric patient. Similarly in medical and surgical wards students need to be reminded about the psychiatric and social aspects of these patients. In some patients an *exclusively* surgical, medical or psychiatric approach can deal with the main problem, but in many patients some sort of *multi-faceted approach* is needed.

The details of history taking will not be repeated here, but students must learn particularly to combine medical and psychiatric history taking. Some common clinical problems for which such a combined medical and psychiatric history are required are:

(1) Patients who have a chronic physical illness (e.g., chronic bronchitis, chronic heart disease, neurological diseases, etc.) should be specifically asked for the presence of depressive symptoms (e.g., sleep disturbance, loss of interest, etc.). If such symptoms are present, specific anti-depressive treatment may be of great value (see chapter 12).

(2) Anxiety, phobic and other neurotic symptoms are frequent in patients who develop a physical illness, particularly if this is an acute severe illness, and the patient previously had been in good health (e.g., cardiac infarction). The significance of the physical illness to the particular patient can only be assessed in the light of the previous personality and the patient's previous experience of the same physical illness (e.g., sudden deaths in colleagues). The attitude of patients, friends and doctor to the physical illness also is an important factor in producing anxiety symptoms. Harmful iatrogenic factors are now more widely recognized than they were, e.g., unnecessary bed rest or restriction of physical activity. In the general hospitals, patients often complain that they are never told why certain tests are done, or what is wrong with them, or how long they will be ill and so on. Residents should explain to every patient, (in terms suitable to the individual) the illness, the investigations, the treatment and the future. Such communications are of great value.

(3) In the elderly, depressive illness often seems to be precipitated by a physical illness (see chapter 16).

Diagnosis and Management

The problems of the diagnosis and management of neurotic and depressive symptoms have been described elsewhere (see chapters 10 and 12).

The treatment of these psychiatric symptoms, even if associated with severe physical illness, may produce great benefit to the patient concerned. It is important to try to assess the relative importance of the psychiatric and physical symptoms so that the total management of the patient can be decided upon. The management of these patients is usually the responsibility of the family doctor, and long term supportive care is most important.

There are certain areas in medicine in which psychiatrists have a particular interest. These include the problems of pain, epilepsy, the care of the dying patient, grief and mourning. The following notes outline some of the psychiatric aspects of these important problems.

PAIN

A common clinical problem is a patient complaining of persistent pain, yet on examination no physical abnormality is found to explain this. These pains are often labelled 'hysterical' or 'functional' and the patient may or may not be referred to a psychiatrist. If referred, the psychiatrist attempts to make a positive diagnosis of psychiatric illness (see chapter 10). Sometimes these patients are found to have depressive symptoms, occasionally they are schizophrenic, and occasionally hysteria *does* seem the appropriate diagnosis. *Most often none of these formal psychiatric labels are strictly appropriate*—certainly theories of hysteria do not account for the pains in most instances. Walters (1969) has reviewed this clinical problem and has suggested classifying 'psychogenic pain' into three main groupings:

(1) Psychogenic magnification of physical pain.

(2) Psychogenic muscular pain (e.g., 'tension' headaches, spastic colon, severe dysmenorrhoea).

(3) Psychogenic regional pain, where there is no peripheral cause for the pain; the pain is regional in site and seems to be related to psychological factors. More women than men present with these symptoms, while age incidence is wide (20-70 years). The pains are usually in the head, over the heart or in the back. This regional distribution is 'unanatomical' with regard to peripheral nerve distribution. The pains are described usually in language of metaphor, e.g., 'my head feels as if it is being squeezed in a vice.' The usual psychiatric diagnoses made in these patients are depression, anxiety or hysteria. Theoretical explanations of how these pains are produced are still incomplete; some authorities liken them to somatic hallucinations.

Investigation and Management

The investigation of these patients should be a *total* search for physical, psychiatric and social factors with a complete history (from both patient and relatives), as well as all the necessary ancillary investigations. The management of neurotic and depressive symptoms has been discussed elsewhere. It should be emphasized that anti-depressive medication is often worth a therapeutic trial in some patients with persistent psychogenic regional pain, even in the absence of marked depressive symptoms, imipramine (Tofranil) being the drug of choice.

EPILEPSY

Recent work has shown that the most useful classifications of epilepsy depend on the fact that some seizures originate in the cerebral cortex itself and others in subcortical structures. Most patients with focal cortical epilepsy have some local structural changes affecting the cortex, while patients whose seizures arise from subcortical structures have either diffuse cerebral damage or none at all.

Disorders Directly Associated with an Epileptic Attack

The Aura

In focal cortical epilepsy the patient's account of the aura of the fit can lead to a knowledge of its site of origin. The complex and variable 'auras' described by patients whose seizures arise in focal cortical areas of the temporal lobe (or adjacent areas) are of great interest to psychiatrists as they have similarities to many symptoms seen in the so called 'functional' group of psychiatric illnesses. These symptoms include unusual epigastric sensations; emotional experiences—fear, anger, depression and pleasure; and hallucinations of one or more modality. Auditory hallucinations are of sounds—music or words. Visual hallucinations may be of stationary or moving objects and there may be micropsia or macropsia. There may also be changes in feelings in parts of the body or the whole body (depersonalization). There may be changes in time appreciation or feelings of familiarity (déjà vu). These complex auras do not last more than a few seconds, though subjectively (as in dreams) they may seem longer. These symptoms may occur alone, be followed by a convulsive fit or by automatism (psychomotor seizure) (see below).

After the Fit

Following the fit there may be periods when there are alterations of consciousness and disturbances in behaviour. These last are greatest after seizures arising in the temporal lobe and may consist of antisocial acts. These behavioural disturbances are confined to a *limited period* immediately after the fit. This time relationship is important because of the possible defence in a court of law that an anti-social act was due to epileptic 'automatism'.

Some epileptics who have had several fits can develop more long lasting behavioural disturbances with paranoid ideas, auditory hallucinations and clouding of consciousness. Abnormal E.E.G. recordings are found during this time.

Disorders not Clearly Associated with an Overt Seizure

A Schizophrenic Syndrome and Temporal Lobe Epilepsy

Chronic paranoid hallucinatory states are known to occur in patients who have had temporal lobe epilepsy for many years. Over the years, the fits diminish in frequency, but a psychiatric syndrome with schizophrenic symptoms develop. The relationships of the similar symptoms seen in schizophrenia proper and temporal lobe functions are, of course, of great interest.

Personality Abnormalities

The majority of epileptics show personality features within the normal range. In about 15% definite abnormalities are found. Physical, psychological and social factors may all contribute towards causing these abnormalities. Some of these patients have severe cerebral damage, and have intellectual deterioration. Others are of normal intelligence and have temporal lobe epilepsy. Abnormal personality features seen in this group of patients include irritability, impulsiveness, stubbornness and aggressive anti-social behaviour. Some of the patients with temporal lobe epilepsy show some of these personality features, while the 'schizophrenic' syndrome, described above, is rare. Again, these personality features cannot be attributed to the seizures alone and they tend to develop as seizures get less frequent.

The problems of the diagnosis and treatment of epilepsy are discussed in textbooks of medicine and will not be described here.

THE DYING PATIENT

The problems of the dying patient are not usually discussed in textbooks of medicine, yet they are most important for all doctors, students and nurses. Instead of making general remarks, attention will be drawn to a book by Hinton (1974) which described the physical discomforts, mental state and personal history of 102 patients dying in hospital (usually from neoplastic conditions), compared with other patients who were suffering from serious but not fatal physical illness. Interviews with these two groups of patients enabled the observer to rate physical distress and strength of religious faith, and the mental state, i.e., depression, anxiety and impairment of consciousness. Awareness of dying was also rated by statements made by patients during their conversation. In addition social and family details were recorded.

As would be expected, the dying had a significantly higher incidence of unrelieved physical distress. They were more commonly depressed (45%) and often anxious (37%). At the first interview Hinton found that half the patients revealed awareness that the illness might be fatal and later 75% thought death probable.

In the last week before death 20% became sure that death was approaching. Depression and anxiety had significant associations with the duration and discomfort of the terminal illness and was more marked in patients under 50.

The implications of this study were that:

(1) Most of the patients were relieved by the opportunity to talk about their feelings and personal problems.

(2) Most dying patients in the last few weeks of their life, realize the fact that they will die—a finding which many doctors deny. The often asked question 'should the doctor tell' hence loses its force.

(3) The mental distress of these patients is significant; its relief by appropriate medication is important (e.g., morphine and allied substances).

Elisabeth Ross (1969) has described a number of 'stages' that are seen in adult dying patients (and their families). The first stage is one of *denial* which may last minutes to months. It is important that this denial is respected.

Then patients become difficult and *angry* and complain especially about family and hospital staff. Patients should be allowed to talk about this anger.

The patient then becomes *depressed,* becoming silent and less interested in his environment.

Finally there is a stage of *acceptance* when he wants to see only a few people close to him and accepts that he will die and gives up any hope of life saving procedures.

This brief discussion on the dying patient leads on to the effects of this on the nearest relatives, again a most important problem for the family doctor.

BEREAVEMENT, GRIEF AND MOURNING

When a love tie is severed, a reaction, emotional and behavioural, is set in train which we call *grief*. The pain of grief is the price we pay for love.

Grief resembles a physical injury. The 'wound' gradually heals, but sometimes complications set in and healing is delayed. Healing can bring strengths. The characteristic feature of grief is the pining or yearning for the lost love object.

Psychiatrists have been aware for many years of the symptoms that can develop in a bereaved person. Because of the frequency of these reactions in the community, they should be more widely appreciated. A study of 72 London widows by Marris (1958) gives a clear picture of what occurs.

There was a sense of futility with an inability to understand the loss and a need to blame someone. This is often the doctor who looked after the husband. *'Physical' symptoms were universal*—particularly loss of weight, pains in the chest, difficulty in breathing, indigestion, headaches and sleeping difficulties. They became apathetic and were restless at home and tended to wander about the streets and parks. They could not believe that their husband was dead and clung to his possessions. There was a tendency to withdraw from friends and relatives.

These symptoms of 'grief' were accepted as natural, but in successful mourning the conflicts of grief were resolved. Freud showed that mourning is a complex task, during which time the bereaved person slowly accustoms himself to the loss of the loved person. While it is going on, the world at large loses its interest. If this does not occur the above symptoms persist and *morbid grief* occurs. The needs of the children are the greatest incentive to master grief, but symptoms only gradually abate. 'You never really get over it' was a typical comment in the study mentioned.

The usual stages of bereavement are that, in the initial phase there is a brief period of shock, numbness and disbelief. Then follows a time of intense pining and yearning, with a sense of protest and resentment. Then over the weeks, the reality of the loss produces sadness, despair and hopelessness. Anger and guilt feelings are important at this time and it is important that the bereaved person has an opportunity to express these feelings. Gradually these feelings pass and the bereaved person begins to look to the outside world and make new relationships.

Why does grief resolve spontaneously in the course of a few months, in some, while in other people symptoms of various sorts persist as an 'abnormal grief reaction'? This is an important question not easily answered. Often patients who develop an abnormal grief reaction have been unusually dependent on the dead person, and may be shy, timid people. Another important factor is a relationship in which both love and hate are prominent and the survivor feels guilty about the death. More abnormal grief reactions may follow unexpected deaths, while previous exposure to death in childhood (of parents or siblings) are also important factors.

Studies in general practice have shown that widows see their family doctor for psychiatric symptoms at three times the usual rate in the first six months after bereavement. The consultation rate for non-psychiatric symptoms also is increased by nearly half. Many of these 'physical' symptoms were referred to the joints or muscles.

Bereavement carries a considerably increased risk of mortality, particularly in men.

Death of a loved person can be followed by:

(1) A 'normal' grief reaction—symptoms lasting several months.
(2) An 'abnormal' grief reaction—with severe long lasting symptoms of the type described above. This is essentially a variety of depressive illness.
(3) Somatic symptoms particularly of joints and muscles may be particularly prominent as part of (2).
(4) Psychosomatic illnesses particularly ulcerative colitis, asthma, peptic ulceration.
(5) Neurotic symptoms can predominate, particularly depersonalization and phobias.
(6) Alcoholism can develop, or if present, become worse after a bereavement.

(7) Other psychiatric illnesses can develop after bereavement (e.g., mania). Usually these patients have had similar illnesses previously.

Prevention and Treatment

Treatment should if possible start before bereavement—it is important for doctors to see that the relatives of a seriously ill person are aware of his approaching death.

Generally, inhibition of grief tends to prolong and complicate mourning and it is not helpful to encourage the bereaved to try and forget their loss. The extremity of grief is dulled over the years, though anniversaries can cause a flare up of symptoms.

The mourning process is an essential part of resolving loss; it is an intensely emotional remembering. Weeping, anger, guilt and sad pleasure may accompany these memories. There is a need to share these feelings and the bereaved person must be allowed to do so. When the patient is unable to weep or be angry or sad, the doctor may need to encourage this grief. Bereavement is an important crisis in a person's life and help at this time (crisis intervention) can be therapeutically valuable.

Supportive care and medication (hypnotics, anti-depressants or tranquillizers) are important in the management of the bereaved patient and the family doctor should accept the fact that *these patients are ill and will need prolonged help*. Psychotherapy for the patient who has severe disabling symptoms may be necessary. The psychotherapist has to encourage the patient to talk about the dead person and particularly to verbalize his hostile feelings.

SUMMARY

In this chapter the importance of physical and psychiatric illnesses occurring together is emphasized. Evaluation and treatment of both illnesses is essential.

Psychogenic regional pain is described and its management discussed.

Some aspects of epilepsy are described.

The problems of the dying patient are discussed.

The effect of bereavement is described and symptoms of abnormal grief reactions are detailed.

REFERENCES

PAIN

Merskey, H. and Spear, F. G., *Pain: psychological and psychiatric aspects.* Baillière, Tindall & Cassell (London, 1967).

Walters, A., 'Psychogenic regional pain alias hysterical pains', *Brain*, 84: 1-18 (1969).

EPILEPSY

Slater, E. and Roth, M., *Clinical Psychiatry*, chapter 8. Baillière, Tindall & Cassell (London, 1969).

DYING, GRIEF AND MOURNING

Bowlby, J., 'Process of mourning', *International Journal of Psychoanalysis*, vol. 42 (1961), p. 317.

Hinton, J. M., *Dying*. Pelican (Harmondsworth, 1974). A book that all medical students should read.

Marris, P., *Widows and their Families*. Routledge & Kegan Paul (London, 1958). A valuable social survey of an important problem.

Parkes, C. M., *Bereavement: studies of grief in adult life*. Tavistock, 1972. A readable overview by an expert.

Ross, E. K., *On Death and Dying*. McMillan (New York, 1969). An important book describing how the author learnt about facing death from her terminally ill patients.

14

PSYCHOSOMATIC MEDICINE

The ill defined area of medicine called 'psychosomatic medicine' was outlined in the 1930s when it was found that certain illnesses could not be explained on completely physical lines. *Illnesses that are included in this field of study are those where a case has been made out for believing that sustained or intense emotional disturbances can play a part in causing, aggravating or maintaining the localized morbid process that is characteristic of the disease in question.* These illnesses include bronchial asthma, peptic ulceration, ulcerative colitis, migraine and certain cardiovascular skin and gynaecological conditions. They are best called 'psychophysiological disorders'.

The development of medicine has produced two separate methodologies: one for studying physical and one for studying psychological phenomena. However the patient is one person, and it is our methods of study that produce the artificial distinction between the physical and psychological. Present methods of medical education make it unusual for one doctor to be able to assess the physical and psychological aspects of the patient on an equal basis. The illnesses considered in this chapter can therefore often usefully be studied by a psychiatrist and physician working together, to assess the causes of the illness and to define the best way of treating the patient.

It has been mentioned in the previous chapter that in everyday clinical practice some illnesses can usually be dealt with by an exclusively physical approach (e.g., most fractures) while in others (e.g., an anxious patient) an exclusively psychiatric approach may be most helpful. This is shown schematically in Figure 1. In such a scheme the psychosomatic group of illnesses fall between these extreme approaches.

Bronchial Asthma

Some general remarks about bronchial asthma will illustrate why this illness is included in the 'psychosomatic group'. It is a common disorder affecting between 1 and 2% of the population and occurring at all ages. Before the age of 14, twice as many boys as girls have asthma, while after 14 the opposite sex difference is found. Two thirds of patients with bronchial asthma give a family history of asthma, hay fever or eczema, showing that there is an important constitutional element present. Bronchial asthma occurs in attacks, and there often are free intervals, sometimes for many years. Between attacks no abnormal physical signs are found in the chest.

Anxious Patient
Psychosomatic illnesses e.g., peptic ulcer, migraine, asthma
Fractures

PHYSICAL APPROACH
Figure 1

Much work has been done on the relationship between allergy and bronchial asthma but unless the concept of 'allergy' is expanded beyond its usual meaning, it does not provide a complete explanation of the cause of most attacks of asthma.

It is helpful to think of the asthmatic, as a person, with stimuli that can cause asthma coming from the 'outer' world—dusts, pollen, bacteria and viruses; and also from his 'inner' world—psychological and endocrine factors are important here.

In general, asthma attacks are precipitated by allergic or infective or psychological factors or by a combination of these factors. Studies which have assessed their importance have shown that 'pure' allergic asthma is the least common, while the commonest problem is the patient with so called intrinsic asthma, in which a combination of infective and psychological factors are important in causing the attacks.

Psychiatric interviews with asthmatics has shown that two sorts of psychological factors can frequently precipitate an attack of bronchial asthma:

(1) Any sudden intense emotion such as rage, fear or sexual feelings.
(2) Any inhibition of emotion e.g., suppression of anger. Because of their personality structure asthmatic patients often have difficulty in expressing their feelings in the usual way.

93

The psychosomatic approach to patients with frequent attacks of bronchial asthma is thus to assess the relative importance of psychological, infective and allergic factors in the particular patient and to suggest appropriate treatment. In order to assess these factors complete medical and psychiatric histories need to be taken along with relevant investigations—e.g., radiographs of chest and sinuses and skin tests.

A similar approach to all the illnesses included in the psychosomatic group is necessary. *The relevance of physical and psychological factors is assessed on an equal basis, so that appropriate treatment may follow.*

Personality and Psychosomatic Illness

One problem that has been widely studied in psychosomatic medicine is the one of the personality characteristics of patients who develop each psychosomatic illness. It has been held that certain types of personality are more likely to develop certain diseases, e.g. the energetic, striving business man has a cardiac infarction, while the lean, restless bus driver gets a duodenal ulcer. Ulcerative colitis is said to be found particularly in obsessional, inhibited people and so on. These conclusions were based on studies of special samples of ulcer or coronary patients, i.e., those patients who attend the teaching hospitals (or an even more special group—those who visit psychoanalysts). Recent studies using objective tests of personality and 'proper' samples of patients have not confirmed these ideas. It is however found that obsessional and other neurotic personality traits are more frequent in patients with psychosomatic illness than in patients with 'pure' organic illnesses.

In addition to studies on the personality features of patients with psychosomatic illnesses, the following important lines of investigation are mentioned in order to illustrate the fact that the 'aetiology' of these illnesses cannot be fully considered by the usual pathological explanations:

Epidemiological studies of psychosomatic illnesses have shown different racial, sex, age and social class distributions as well as seasonal fluctuations. For example, duodenal ulceration is more frequently seen in managers and executives than in other industrial workers. Doctors have a high incidence of duodenal ulceration while a low incidence is found in agricultural workers.

The significance of 'stress' has been shown in studies that investigate social and psychological factors operating at the onset of the illness or at a relapse of symptoms. These studies have clearly shown the relationship of onset of symptoms with 'stress'. In one study, emotional factors seemed important in 84% of 205 ulcer patients admitted to hospital compared with 22% of a control group of hernia patients.

In taking the history from patients it is often useful to tabulate the physical, psychological and social data in a chronological order on a life chart (see Appendix 2) so that these relationships can be seen. In this regard it is important to check on the patient's history—from relatives or hospital records, as it is very easy for the patient to 'telescope' events that are outstanding, so that they may seem to coincide with the onset of symptoms, if the patient's story is accepted without outside verification. One should aim to define the patient's personality and his particular situation at a point in time. Clinically one thinks of an individual in a situation in which anger or depression are evoked, but their expression is suppressed.

Another important group of studies have been those that have studied *the relationship between psychological and somatic events.* The model for these studies are the experiments of Wolff and Wolf on their subject Tom who had a gastric fistula. These workers studied gastric function by assessing the vascularity of the stomach mucosa and the stomach acidity. Changes observed were correlated with changes in Tom's emotions. They employed Tom in their laboratory and so were able to understand his personality, and also to be aware of any problems at work or in his domestic life. They found that Tom's stomach blanched with fear and depression while the acid secretion fell. Aggression, resentment and anxiety produced vascular engorgement and an increase in acid secretion. Under these conditions the stomach mucosa was prone to ulceration. These studies draw attention to the fact that clinically, in patients with peptic ulceration one cannot consider the ulcer in isolation from the patient as a person reacting in his own way to his unique environment.

Studies in depth of patients with psychosomatic illnesses by psychotherapists have given valuable information about the personality structure of these particular patients. Other studies of the families of young men with peptic ulcers have given interesting information about the family relationships of these subjects. As has been mentioned generalizations from these limited studies should not be made.

TREATMENT

Even if emotional factors are shown to be important in producing symptoms in a particular patient, this does not mean that the best, i.e. most effective, treatment is psychotherapy, unaccompanied by other treatments.

In fact the value of formal psychotherapy in these disorders is limited. What is important however, in everyday clinical practice, is that along with some medical regime, e.g. diet and alkalis in peptic ulceration, or antispasmodics and antibiotics in asthma, the patient is also considered from the psychiatric and social viewpoints and the principles of supportive care (chapter 9) applied. In particular when seeing these patients regularly, in general or private practice, discussion should move from the symptoms to the patient's interpersonal problems at home and at work. In particular the patient should learn greater freedom of emotional expression, while relaxation methods may also be helpful.

In theory there are a number of 'levels' at which treatment can be directed. Taking peptic ulceration as an example we can consider:

THE PATIENT	POSSIBLE TREATMENT
environment	social changes
patient as a person	psychotherapy
brain function	drug treatment (e.g. sedatives, tranquillizers), leucotomy
vagus nerve	vagotomy, anticholinergic drugs
stomach (end organ)	antacids, diet, surgery

In most patients several of these approaches may be used.

CLINICAL EXAMINATION

J. L. Halliday, a pioneer in the study of psychosomatic illness, has suggested certain questions that should be answered during the history taking procedure on a patient with a psychosomatic illness. They are:

(1) *Why did this patient become ill at this time?* All events and situations occurring about the time of onset of the symptoms should be gone into thoroughly. Their significance to the patient can only be judged by assessing his personality, in the way already described, so that the next question:

(2) *What sort of person is this?* can be answered.

(3) *Why did this person develop this illness and not another?*
Often this question cannot be answered fully, but family history and previous symptoms involving a particular system e.g., alimentary canal, chest are important. After the patient has improved it is worth asking oneself:

(4) *Why did this patient get better at this time?* As these patients often have recurrent attacks of symptoms (peptic ulcer, asthma), it may be helpful for the future management of the patient to try to answer this question.

SUMMARY

Psychosomatic illnesses are those in which sustained or intense emotional disturbances play a part in causing, aggravating or maintaining the localized morbid process that is characteristic of the disease in question.

Using bronchial asthma as an example, the psychosomatic approach which investigates the physical, psychiatric and social aspects of the patient on an equal basis is illustrated.

Some of the main areas of research in psychosomatic medicine are outlined.

Certain useful clinical questions to ask in patients with these illnesses are detailed.

REFERENCES

Hamilton, M., *Psychosomatics*. Chapman & Hall (London, 1955). A brief, balanced account of all aspects of the subject.

Leigh, D., 'Recent advances in psychosomatic medicine', *Med. J. Aust.*, i: 327 (1968).

Meares, R., 'A model of psychosomatic illness', *Medical Journal of Australia*, vol. 2, (1975), p. 97.

Munro, A., *Psychosomatic Medicine*. Churchill (Livingstone, 1973). A small paperback containing papers published in the *Practitioner*.

Wolff, H. C. and Wolf, S., *Human Gastric Function*. Oxford University Press, 1947. The classic monograph in psychosomatic medicine.

15

ACUTE AND CHRONIC BRAIN SYNDROMES

It has previously been mentioned that in the present state of our knowledge psychiatric syndromes are divided into an *organic* group in which brain pathology can be shown to exist by present techniques and a *functional* group where no such pathology can be shown.

Organic brain syndromes are separated clinically from functional syndromes by the presence of *memory disturbances* and varying degrees of *clouding of consciousness*. This last symptom complex varies in severity, but essentially the patient is not in full contact with his temporal and spatial environment, so that he is disorientated in time and place.

Organic syndromes can be divided into two large groups: the *acute brain syndrome* (delirium) which is completely reversible and the *chronic brain syndrome* which is not, and leads to a permanent and irreversible decline of all mental abilities (dementia). Sometimes the two syndromes are combined. A *subacute brain syndrome* is occasionally a useful clinical diagnosis.

Aetiology

The causes of these brain syndromes cannot be deduced from an examination of the mental state alone, e.g., the mental states of patients with a cerebral tumour or general paralysis of the insane or chronic alcoholism may be identical. The separation of the causes of these illnesses therefore depends upon a full medical and psychiatric history and a complete medical examination with appropriate ancillary investigations. It is also important to recognize that the psychiatric symptoms present in both these syndromes are 'shaped' by the patient's previous personality and his previous psychiatric health.

Both these syndromes can result from traumatic, toxic, metabolic, infective, neoplastic or degenerative factors but it will be convenient to describe these syndromes separately.

ACUTE BRAIN SYNDROME (Delirium or Confusional State)

Aetiology

This syndrome is due to some acute disturbances in cerebral tissue functioning. These disturbances may be due to

(a) oxygen lack
(b) glucose lack
(c) breakdown of enzyme systems related to carbohydrate or amino acid metabolism
(d) presence of toxic substances (e.g., ammonia, urea)
(e) a combination of these factors.

Clinically the usual causes of the acute brain syndrome can be grouped as:

Infective

Infections at any age, *but particularly in the old and young*. These infections may be generalized, e.g., the specific fevers of childhood, or may be localized (particularly in the chest and kidneys). Infections of the central nervous system are another important group of conditions causing this syndrome.

Toxic

Alcohol and drugs are the important toxic factors. Most drugs in *excessive amounts* will produce this syndrome but the following are the ones most frequently encountered clinically: barbiturates and other sedative drugs (including bromides), insulin, steroids, amphetamines, atropine, anti-parkinsonian drugs, isoniazid, anti-convulsants.

Withdrawal of alcohol or barbiturates is a common cause of this syndrome.

Metabolic Causes

Cardiac failure (acute or chronic). Hypoglycaemia and hyperglycaemia; liver and renal failure (often secondary to prostatic disease in the elderly man). Disorders of the thyroid gland. Vitamin deficiency.

Traumatic

Post-epileptic states. Brain injury.

One of the commonest presentations of this syndrome is after operations where a number of aetiological factors may be present. Elderly patients and alcoholics are particularly liable to develop the acute brain syndrome post-operatively.

Clinical Features

Perhaps the most important clinical feature is the *fluctuating severity* of the symptoms, which are often worse at night. Because of this fluctuation, different observers, or the same observer at different times may report—and be puzzled by—quite contrasting behaviour and memory function.

There is a *clouding of consciousness* so that the patient is not fully aware of outside events, and on questioning shows varying degrees of disorientation in time and place. The patient is often *restless*—particularly at night—and again this symptom can vary in severity. The combination of *disorientation* and *restlessness* is called *confusion*.

Visual hallucinations in the setting of clouding of consciousness are characteristic of the more severe types of acute brain syndrome (e.g., delirium tremens).

Even in mild cases, *anxiety* is a common symptom, but extreme fear can be seen, particularly in association with visual hallucinations.

Thinking is disturbed; often thoughts are rapid and chaotic, and fleeting delusions may be seen.

Occasionally the patient repeats well established tasks giving rise to an 'occupational delirium'. Words and phrases may be repeated over and over again by the patient.

The *duration of the symptoms* may be overnight (as is often the case with a young febrile child) or days or weeks in more severe cases. The course of the illness is usually towards recovery and rarely lasts longer than a month.

Methods of Study

It is particularly important to discover the causative factors by full physical examinations and investigations.

From the point of view of noting progress of the mental state it is useful to *record verbatim* every few days the patient's answers to the same questions on orientation (see Appendix 3).

Prevention

Operations in the elderly and alcoholics are liable to be followed by these symptoms. Pre- and post-operative attention should therefore be full and particular care taken with eye operations in the elderly.

Treatment

The essential of treatment is to identify and treat the aetiological factors involved.

Patients with an acute brain syndrome should be nursed in a quiet room with constant lighting throwing a minimum of shadows. Experienced nursing is particularly valuable throughout the 24 hours. Correction of dehydration is important and extra fluids need to be given orally (or intravenously if necessary). Electrolyte control may be important.

Infections are the usual causes of this syndrome and need specific treatment. In this regard, infections in elderly patients may be difficult to define and treatment may have to be given empirically.

In severe cases the patient will be helped by tranquillizing drugs, e.g., chlorpromazine (Largactil) 100 mg. q.d.s. or thiordazine (Melleril) 100 mg. q.d.s. It is better to use these drugs at night as well and not sedatives. Dosage may have to be much increased according to the severity of the symptoms.

It is also worthwhile in these severe cases to give parental vitamin preparations—by intramuscular or intravenous injection daily for 4-5 days—followed by oral preparations. The injections should contain a minimum of 100 mg. of aneurine hydrochloride and 160 mg. of nicotinamide.

Gradually as the patient improves, the tranquillizing drugs should be reduced, then stopped and the patient's activities and diet increased accordingly.

CHRONIC BRAIN SYNDROME

Aetiology

As has been mentioned, chronic brain syndromes (dementias) are irreversible and progressive. There are however a minority of patients who present *a dementing clinical picture*, but where the causes *are* treatable and the patient's clinical state can improve. It is therefore important in every patient who appears 'demented' to consider whether the following could be present:

(1) cerebral syphilis
(2) a cerebral tumour
(3) a subdural haematoma
(4) myxoedema
(5) pernicious anaemia
(6) vascular lesions, which also need careful investigation in view of advancing medical and surgical knowledge
(7) normal pressure hydrocephalus. In this condition the P.E.G. shows dilation of the entire ventricular system. An arachnoiditis causes obstruction at the foramina of Magendie and Lushka. Clinically there may be dementia, retardation, gait disorder and urinary incontinence. Surgical treatment can be helpful.

In general however, the causes of the chronic brain syndromes may be grouped as:

Degenerative

Here there is a primary 'idiopathic' degeneration of cortical cells. Such conditions include senile dementia, and the presenile group which comprises Alzheimer's and Pick's disease (a progressive dementia with focal signs), as well as Huntington's chorea and disseminated sclerosis.

Vascular

The syndrome may result from cerebro-vascular accidents producing multiple cerebral infarctions or haemorrhage. Hypertension is also an important factor to be considered.

Toxic Factors

Alcohol producing Korsakoff's syndrome or alcoholic dementia.

Traumatic

Severe brain injury; punch drunkenness.

Tumour

Primary or secondary intracranial neoplasms.

Metabolic

Hypothyroid states (cretinism or myxoedema).
    Vit. B_{12} deficiency
    Vit. B_2 deficiency (pellagra).
    Prolonged oxygen deprivation (as after carbon monoxide poisoning or post anaesthetic).

Infective
Syphilis.

Congenital
The clinical features of the congenital chronic brain syndrome (severe mental retardation) will not be detailed here.

Pathology
Only some general points of clinical importance will be mentioned. At post mortem, differentiation between the various types of disorders may be impossible. In 20% of elderly dements, senile and arteriosclerotic processes are found together.

Pathologically any histological distinction between senile dementia and Alzheimer's disease may not be valid; while clinically the separation of Pick's and Alzheimer's disease is unreliable.

Psychopathology
Explanation of the behaviour of patients with a chronic organic brain syndrome usually follows the ideas of Hughlings Jackson. He interpreted some symptoms as being *negative* in the sense that they were directly due to loss of function. Others were called *positive* symptoms because they were 'released' when higher controls were abolished by the disease process. In addition Jackson emphasized that complex skills are lost first, while the more automatic the action, the longer it is unaffected by the degenerative process.

The way the patients adapt to waning intellectual powers is important. They learn to avoid tasks they know they cannot do, and live a much more regularized life, which if disturbed can produce outbursts of anger or weeping. In this respect it has been shown that dementing patients who previously had a 'difficult' personality are more likely to be admitted to a psychiatric hospital, while other dementing patients can be managed at home by their families.

Clinical Features
The central such feature is *impaired memory*. Recently-acquired memories are lost before memories established in the remote past (Ribot's Law). The patient becomes unable to retain or recall recent impressions. The first important sign of this in examining the mental state is the patient's inability to recall facts about current events (e.g., name of the President of the U.S.A., Prime Minister of Britain, etc.). Questions about memory should follow a regular scheme as suggested in Appendix 3. In everyday life this memory impairment is compensated for by the patient restricting his interests, by following a rigid timetable and often the use of a notebook.

A *poverty of thought* develops along with *impaired judgment* and *reasoning*. A business man may show these abnormalities by a failure to grasp the meaning of some event at work and making some grossly inept remarks.

The *mood* of most patients is profoundly altered. Irritability, euphoria and lability of mood are among the earliest changes. Weeping over trifles is common. Some patients experience persistent depressive symptoms. Gradually *apathy* and *indifference* develop as the main features of the patient's mood.

Delusions occur as a result of the disturbances in reasoning and emotions. They are characteristically unorganized and transitory and usually grandiose, paranoid or hypochondriacal. Ideas of being robbed are particularly frequent—often subsequent to the patient losing some object because of his memory difficulty.

Care of personal appearance, mode of dressing, eating, and personal habits all gradually deteriorate.

The syndrome of dementia usually indicates the presence of diffuse cerebral disease. Local involvement can give rise to focal symptoms—fits, speech disturbances, apraxias, etc., that are seen as part of the clinical picture in these patients.

Course of the Illness

This is usually a steady progressive deterioration and death follows usually within a few years. There can be episodic fluctuations, particularly in arteriosclerotic dementia.

Methods of Study

It has been emphasized that a full medical, psychiatric and social history needs to be taken from the patient and the relatives, and a full physical examination carried out along with all necessary ancillary investigations necessary to define the cause of the condition. *A global diagnosis of dementia is not sufficient.*

As regards the mental state it is useful to define memory impairment firstly along simple clinical lines and also by more formal psychological testing. Repeated testing may be a useful guide to the progress of the disorder. The social effects of the symptoms must also be clearly defined. It is these that cause hospital admission.

Of ancillary investigations, electroencephalography, 'brain scans' with radioisotopes; radiography (computerized axial tomography and arteriography) and occasionally brain biopsy are important in helping to define the cause and extent of the cerebral atrophy (see chapter 16).

Differential Diagnosis

(1) Depressive illness: Elderly people with a depressive illness can appear to have memory impairment and dementia. (So called 'pseudodementia'). This is important as treatment for depression is available. A history from the relative is probably the most valuable diagnostic aid, when depressive symptoms should be specifically asked for (see chapter 16).

(2) Senescence: The separation of normal old age and pathological dementia is a complex one. Memory impairment is seen in both groups of patients but the rate of progress of the deterioration is much greater in senile dementia.

Prevention

At present little can be said about preventing senile dementia and arterial disease. Perhaps the main aspect of *treatment* should be preventing, as far as possible, the family and social problems presented by the dementing elderly person in the household, that lead to hospital admissions.

Treatment

Treatable 'dementing' processes have been described—syphilis, tumour, etc., and should never be overlooked.

For the majority of patients, it is a problem of general supportive care by the family doctor. He has to help the patient, and also help the family to cope with the problems presented by the gradually deteriorating dement, and this is not an easy task. As has been mentioned if the patient's previous personality has been 'difficult' then behavioural problems are more likely.

In addition to the consequences of the memory impairment the development of *paranoid* and *depressive* symptoms are important to recognize and treat. Paranoid symptoms respond to phenothiazine drugs, e.g. chlorpromazine (Largactil) 50-100 mg. t.d.s., or trifluoperazine (Stelazine) 5-20 mg. nocte.

Depressive symptoms should be treated with imipramine (Tofranil) 75-300 mg. per day or similar drug (see chapter 12).

Regular activities are important for the dementing patient, and interests should be encouraged for as long as possible. Day Centres are available in some places and help patients and relatives.

Demented patients are often particularly restless at night when they become more disorientated. Even in the absence of paranoid symptoms, regular treatment with phenothiazine drugs is often helpful for these nocturnal problems, e.g. chlorpromazine (Largactil) 50-100 mg. nocte.

Medical care of the heart, lungs and kidney disease etc. should never be neglected.

Admission to hospital depends on social criteria and not strictly medical ones. Relatives' tolerance for demanding patients varies enormously. The effect of the dementia on eating, bowel and bladder habits is important in this regard.

Death usually follows an intercurrent infection—with the development of an acute brain syndrome to complicate the psychiatric picture.

SUMMARY

The acute and chronic brain syndromes are described: their causes and treatment outlined.

The influence of the patient's personality on the presentation of both these syndromes is important.

Tranquillizing drugs and social measures are important in the treatment of chronic brain syndromes: hospital admission should be deferred as long as possible.

Some patients appear to have a chronic brain syndrome, yet the causes are treatable. This small group should not be forgotten.

REFERENCE

Blackwood, W., *Greenfield's Neuropathology*. 3rd edn, Edward Arnold (London, 1976). The standard reference book on this subject.

16

PSYCHIATRIC SYNDROMES IN THE ELDERLY

Psychiatric illnesses are an important part of medical problems in the elderly. Longevity brings an increased expectancy of mental illness and a rising incidence of suicide. Socially isolated and physically handicapped elderly people are particularly liable to psychiatric illness. Already, in psychiatric hospitals, patients over 60 are a more numerous group than young patients with schizophrenia. The general approach to these illnesses however is to establish a diagnosis and treat the patient in the community. Here one of the roles of the family doctor (with out-patient help if needed) is to avoid hospital admission if at all possible.

There are a number of separate psychiatric syndromes seen in the elderly that have contrasting outlooks, and for some of which active treatment is now available. *Labels such as 'senility' or 'dementia' are not satisfactory diagnoses.* The main clinical problems are:

(1) Depressive illness, its treatment and its separation from the chronic brain syndrome.
(2) The management of patients with a chronic brain syndrome.
(3) The identification and treatment of the acute and subacute brain syndromes.
(4) The causes and management of paranoid symptoms in the elderly.
(5) Personality problems and neurosis in the elderly.

METHODS OF STUDY

The History

History must be full and include information about the patient's physical, psychological and social life. Additional histories from the patient's relatives are of particular value in elderly patients.

The *mode of onset* and *duration* of the main symptoms are important as is the *rate of progress* of the disorder. In patients with a long standing illness one should always endeavour to find out why the patient has sought medical help at this time, and here family attitudes to the patient and his illness may be of the greatest importance.

Physical Examination

This must be thorough, and in particular the presence of cardiac, renal or hepatic insufficiency should be carefully assessed. Other toxic factors that can produce psychiatric symptoms are infections that can be difficult to find evidence for in the elderly and here examination of the lungs and renal tract are particularly important.

Diabetes mellitus, myxoedema and anaemia should always be looked for specifically, as should any possible dietary deficiencies. Alcoholism should never be forgotten. Neurological abnormalities need careful assessment. In general, fine tremors, localized areflexias and absent vibration sensation are of little clinical importance in the elderly.

Mental Assessment

This should follow the methods previously defined. In particular assessment of *mood* and *thought content* need careful attention. 'How have you been feeling in yourself lately?' 'Have you lost interest in things?' 'Have you felt life is not worth living?' All these questions must be asked as they give valuable information about the patient's mood.

Perhaps it is in assessing 'memory' clinically that most errors are made. This cannot be done by asking elderly patients arithmetical questions (such as serial sevens or monetary sums). Elderly people vary widely in their ability to do these sorts of tests, so that the effects of illness cannot be judged by their answers.

The first signs of memory impairment in patients with a dementing illness are to be found in their answers to questions about recent world events. Therefore simple tests such as: 'Can you tell me the name of the President of the United States?' 'How long has he been President?' 'When did the last war start and finish?' should be used. Gross errors in replies to these questions in our society are not explainable by the patient saying he does not know, as he does not read the papers or listen to the wireless, and usually point to the presence of definite memory impairment. It is important however to note that some patients with a depressive illness who are agitated or retarded cannot concentrate and may make quite gross errors even on these simple tests. It is best to approach these tests in a formal order. Questions usually asked are listed in Appendix 3.

It is important for students to recognize that 'organic' patients may confabulate or make facile excuses for not knowing an answer to a simple question. Depressed patients may also not answer correctly but may do so by saying 'I don't know—I can't concentrate!' This *qualitative* difference is an important one in clinical practice. The responses to these questions cannot therefore be scored and used as a quantitative test of memory impairment.

Special Tests (for the clinical problem ?dementia)

These are usually considered when one tries to sort out whether an elderly patient's symptoms are associated with organic brain disease or not. Clinically it may be often best to treat the present symptoms and allow response to treatment and subsequent follow up answer this question.

Psychological Testing

Formal psychological testing is sometimes of value; but if the clinician cannot decide 'organic or functional?' neither can the psychologist. Psychologists can however usefully define memory impairment in response to set tests so that a base line can be obtained, against which progress can be judged.

Computerized axial tomography

An important advance in radiological techniques and is now the most important investigation in these patients.

Electro-encephalography

Severe dementias are usually associated with definite E.E.G. abnormalities but again, in the difficult cases of early dementia then E.E.G. studies are usually of little help. The presence of focal abnormalities and the progress of the condition can however be investigated by serial E.E.G. studies.

Pneumoencephalography (P.E.G.)

This is an unpleasant experience and it is best restricted to patients in whom a space-occupying lesion is suspected. Nevertheless, a significant correlation exists between radiological atrophy as shown by P.E.G. and clinical ratings of dementia.

Cerebral Angiography

This investigation may give valuable information in patients with vascular disease or tumours, but it is not usually contemplated unless surgical intervention is being considered.

Brain Scanning

Intravenous Tc^{99m} is given. This substance does not penetrate the blood-brain barrier unless cerebral pathology is present. This investigation gives information about space-occupying lesions.

Brain Biopsy

This method of investigation at present is used only rarely.

CLINICAL SYNDROMES IN THE ELDERLY

It will be useful to briefly highlight some of the clinical features and problems that these syndromes present in the elderly.

Mood Disorders

(1) *Manic* illnesses are uncommon and will not be described other than to say that the picture is somewhat different from that seen in young adults, and that the separation from symptoms of an acute brain syndrome can be difficult but important.

(2) *Depressive* illnesses are frequent and important because of the risk of suicide and the effectiveness of treatment. In mild cases, with

which the general practitioner is concerned, the association with chronic physical ill health is an important one and it must again be emphasized that depressive symptoms (see chapter 12) must be specifically asked for.

The more severe depressive illnesses that reach hospital often seem to follow (days, weeks or months) some important events—e.g., physical illness, bereavement, serious illness of spouse, children leaving, retirement, moving house. Sometimes these patients have had attacks of depression when they were younger, more often this is not the case. More frequent is the finding in these depressed patients of life long neurotic personality traits—particularly obsessional or phobic symptoms and sexual disinterest.

Over half of these depressed patients present with physical complaints often of a hypochondriacal nature, and it is important not to overlook the depression and continue to investigate the patient for physical disease. Yet other depressed patients do have real physical illness often of a chronic nature, and these patients, as has been mentioned, have a high suicide rate.

Follow up studies have shown that depressive illness in the elderly is not the prodroma of deteriorating organic illness and is unrelated to senile or arteriosclerotic dementia; the prognosis is quite different.

Treatment of depressive illness need not be considered again (see chapter 12) but the value of anti-depressive drugs in this age group is great.

Prognosis of depressive illness in the elderly is generally good, but psychological and social invalidism are long term problems in about half of the patients.

Chronic Brain Syndrome

The causes, symptoms, signs and management of dementing illnesses have been described elsewhere (chapter 15). The cause of a dementia in the elderly is usually a senile or arteriosclerotic process, but the other causes must not be forgotten.

Arteriosclerotic dementia (multi infarct dementia) is characterized by a progressive history of strokes, often hypertension and the presence of focal brain damage, e.g., hemiplegia, dysphasic symptoms. In the absence of this evidence of focal damage, senile dementia with a relentlessly progressive course is more likely. At post mortem, senile and arteriosclerotic processes are often found together. It seems likely that senile dementia is a circumscribed disease and not one extreme of ageing mental processes.

Acute Brain Syndrome

The causes, symptoms, signs and management of this condition have been described (chapter 15). In the elderly the condition is sometimes termed senile delirium or senile confusional state and is particularly liable to follow anaesthetics and operations (note blindfolding in ophthalmic operations).

Often too, the acute confusional state occurs in a patient with a well advanced dementia and is precipitated by some intercurrent physical disease.

Paranoid States

Paranoid symptoms in the elderly are common and they can be symptomatic of a number of different conditions. The word paranoid is used clinically to describe persecutory ideas. These can vary, from patients who have always felt people were hostile to them, to others who have firmly fixed persecutory delusions, perhaps towards a particular person or group of people (e.g., police, freemasons, communists).

Paranoid experiences are frequent in immigrants and partially deaf people.

In general paranoid symptoms are seen in:
(1) depressive illness
(2) acute and chronic brain syndromes
(3) schizophrenia
(4) paranoid personality development (see later).
(1) and (2) will not be described again.

The volitional and affective changes that are the important features of schizophrenic illnesses in earlier life are not prominent in schizophrenia of the elderly. Outside the paranoid experiences, patients may function reasonably well. The mental state is characterized by *delusional ideas* and *hallucinatory phenomena*. The previous personality of about 50% of patients shows prominent traits of suspiciousness, eccentricity, emotional coldness and solitariness.

As a rule paranoid symptoms respond well to tranquillizing drugs whatever the cause of the paranoid symptoms.

For paranoid schizophrenia in the elderly *prolonged* administration of, e.g. trifluoperazine (Stelazine) 10-20 mg. nocte (with an anti-parkinsonian drug, e.g. orphenadrine hydrochloride (Dispal) 50 mg. nocte) often has a profound effect on the delusions and hallucinations, and the way the patient describes and reacts to them. This medication will have to be continued indefinitely in most patients.

Personality Disorders and Neurosis in the Elderly

Clinical experience gives the impression that the personality disorders seen in adolescence and young adult life get less severe with rising age. However there is a definite group of patients, who, with advancing age, develop personality changes—these changes are often exaggerations of minor peculiarities, e.g. patients who become more withdrawn from others, and have a gloomy worrying outlook towards life in general and their own health in particular. These people become more hypochondriacal and more miserly as they age. Others develop paranoid ideas that affect all the various aspects of the patient's life.

Actual neurotic symptoms in the elderly—e.g. anxiety, phobic, obsessional, hysterical and mild depressive symptoms—are more frequent than is usually recorded. While some of these patients may give a life long history of similar neurotic symptoms, others will present with these symptoms for the first time in late life. In these patients any degree of organic deterioration must be assessed and the history carefully taken for the presence of a mild depressive illness. This last is often present and treatment with anti-depressive medication is the most useful pharmacological approach to these patients; though long term supportive care by an interested doctor is the mainstay of medical treatment.

SUMMARY

Psychiatric symptoms in the elderly are an important part of present day medical practice.

A total—physical, psychiatric and social—approach is emphasized.

It is important to separate the main psychiatric syndrome present i.e., acute and chronic brain syndromes, paranoid states, depressive illness and neurosis.

Symptomatic treatment (e.g., particularly of depressive or paranoid symptoms) is important.

Depressive illness in the elderly is emphasized because of its frequency, its presentation (physical symptoms and hypochondriasis) and because it can be actively treated.

REFERENCE

Post, F., *The Clinical Psychiatry of Late Life*. Pergamon Press (Oxford, 1965). An excellent account of the clinical problems of psychiatric illness in the elderly.

17

ALCOHOLISM AND DRUG DEPENDENCE

Alcoholism is a common condition in which the patient's drinking habits are damaging his mental, physical or social health. Some sort of frame of reference is helpful in considering the problems of alcoholism.

Some people are teetotal; others drink at social occasions, and from time to time may get drunk; these are *social drinkers.*

Some people are *excessive drinkers;* they drink frequently, often during the course of their daily work, and social and medical problems may arise. Many of these heavy drinkers can however give up alcohol completely for a while without developing withdrawal symptoms. Most of these people however become *alcohol addicts* who are unable to give up drinking; if they do, withdrawal symptoms occur.

Once the stage is reached where alcohol has produced physical damage to the liver, stomach, nervous system or other organs, the condition is called *chronic alcoholism* (see page 219).

While a number of 'classical hospital' syndromes of mental or physical impairment due to alcohol will be described briefly, it is important to realize that the *real problem is the treatment of the alcoholic before these syndromes develop.* The family doctor gets to know about these early cases in various ways, but often these patients do not readily accept medical advice, although treatment at this stage would be most helpful, e.g. before cirrhosis of the liver develops. Most alcoholics are in fact untreated and unrecognized. It is estimated that 15% of the morbidity in general hospitals is associated with alcohol.

Aetiology

Alcoholism is an important medical and social problem in most countries, and has always been so. Aetiological considerations involved are *social factors, personality factors,* and *chemical dependence.*

There is no evidence that the future alcoholic is different from his fellows as regards physiology and metabolism. Allergy, nutritional or endocrine factors play no part in aetiology. Alcoholism is a familial condition being passed on by example, not by genetic inheritance.

Social and cultural factors determine the incidence of alcoholism in a community, but they act on all its members, though only a small proportion become alcoholics. Full employment, high wages, ample leisure time are important as is the availability and cost of alcohol. Alcoholism is an occupational hazard in those workers who come into the closest contact with alcohol, i.e., publicans, barmen, waiters, brewers, distillers, draymen. Service officers and commercial travellers also have a high alcoholism rate.

As will be mentioned alcoholism usually begins as social drinking and many people start drinking because of their need for company. There is no circumscribed personality of people who become alcoholics. Some alcoholics seem to be closely bound to one or other of their parents and are unable to make a close relationship with anyone else. Other alcoholics give a history of life long sexual problems; still others cannot cope with the 'stress' of everyday living without the relief that alcohol provides. Sometimes alcoholism follows misfortune, e.g. bereavement (death of a child or wife); sometimes alcohol is used by the patient to blunt persistent depressive or neurotic symptoms. Once alcohol is taken regularly, physical dependence may develop, and a vicious circle starts.

SYMPTOMS AND SIGNS OF ALCOHOLISM

Jellinek as a result of detailed investigation formulated his concepts of phases in the drinking history of alcoholics. These are useful in clinical practice and are outlined below:

Prealcoholic Asymptomatic Phase

Alcohol is first used socially, and the prospective alcoholic, in contrast to the social drinker, experiences a rewarding relief of tension in the drinking situation. Over the next 6 months or 2 years his tolerance to tension decreases and alcohol is taken daily. There is, however, no overt intoxication and the drinking is not conspicuous to his associates.

The Prodromal Phase

(1) Though drinking, he does not appear intoxicated and will carry on quite complicated activities, though next day he has memory impairment for the events of the previous day.
(2) Surreptitious drinking and preoccupation with alcohol. The alcohol consumption during this phase is heavy but does not lead to overt intoxication. Periods of amnesia increase and this phase ends with—
(3) Loss of control. Now any drink of alcohol leads to a reaction which is felt by the drinker as a physical demand for alcohol. Any social or emotional conflict causes a renewal of the drinking.

Crucial Phase

At this stage the alcoholic, once started on a bout of drinking, cannot control the amount he will drink, though there can be periods of voluntary abstinence. Alcoholic alibis begin at this stage, and now his drinking behaviour becomes conspicuous to his relatives and employers.

At this time begins the behaviour that stems from the alcoholic's rationalization that the faults lie in others and not in himself.

At this stage there are episodes of marked aggressive behaviour followed by periods of remorse. The hostility towards his environment

113

is associated with his losing jobs and dropping friends. His entire behaviour becomes alcohol centred and he becomes more isolated. Under the impact of these events family problems become more prominent. There is also a decrease in sexual drive which increases hostility towards his wife and gives rise to the alcoholic jealousy syndrome. At this time alcohol is taken as soon as he gets up, and drinking increases as he enters the chronic phase.

Chronic Phase

Here the period of prolonged intoxication begins, with marked ethical deterioration. At this time he drinks with anyone and may begin drinking methylated spirits or cheap wines. Tremors become persistent and these can only be controlled by taking more alcohol. It is at this stage that the alcoholic can admit defeat and seek treatment himself.

In general by the time an alcoholic comes to medical attention there will have been about 8 years of excessive drinking followed by 8 years of alcohol addiction.

ALCOHOL DEPENDENCE

Edwards and Goss have defined the clinical syndrome of alcohol dependence: *British Medical Journal*, vol. 1, no. 6017 (1976), pp. 1058–1061. Essential features of the syndrome are:—

(1) *Narrowing of the drinking repertoire*

As dependence advances, cues related to avoidance of alcohol withdrawal are important and the person's drinking repertoire narrows. The drinking pattern becomes the same on work days, week-ends and holidays. Later the drinking can become a regular daily time-table to maintain a high blood alcohol.

(2) *Salience of drink-seeking behaviour*

Priority is given to maintaining alcohol intake. The wife's distress has less effect, money is used more and more for drink. Physical problems are ignored for drink-seeking behaviour.

(3) *Increased tolerance to alcohol*

The dependant person is able to sustain a high alcohol intake and go about his business with alcohol blood levels that would incapacitate the non-dependant drinker. Patients will say 'I have a good head for it'. Later, for reasons that are unclear, this tolerance is lost.

(4) *Repeated withdrawal symptoms*

In the fully developed picture, the patient wakes with multiple symptoms. Tremors, nausea, sweating and mood disturbances are the key symptoms of withdrawal.

(5) *Relief of withdrawal symptoms by further drinking*

Relief drinking for early cues become important. Early morning drinking becomes a regular clinical feature.

(6) *Subjective awareness of compulsions to drink*

There is a compulsion to drink, a desire to drink more which is seen as irrational but cannot be resisted.

(7) *Reinstatement after abstinence*

Abstinence is often easy in the ward where cues for drinking are removed, but relapse to the previous stage of the dependence syndrome follows. A syndrome that takes years to develop can be fully reinstated after restarting drinking for a few days.

Physical, psychiatric and social disabilities accumulate for the alcohol dependent person, though an individual patient can develop cirrhosis, lose his job, crash his car, and break up his marriage without suffering from the dependence syndrome. Not every person who drinks too much is alcohol dependent.

PSYCHIATRIC DISTURBANCES

(1) *Depressive Symptoms*

The commonest psychiatric symptoms in alcoholics are depressive ones. These are important as alcoholics have a high suicide rate (see chapter 18).

(2) *Acute Intoxication*

The picture of acute intoxication is well known and need not be described here.

(3) *Personality Deterioration*

The personality changes seen in the alcoholic have been described in the previous section (note particularly the periods of brief amnesia and pathological jealousy).

(4) *Withdrawal Syndromes*

Certain syndromes are associated with the absolute or relative withdrawal of alcohol in alcoholics. They are not nutritional in origin as they occur in patients taking normal diets. They are often precipitated by the development of some other event, e.g., an illness like influenza, or post-operatively, when the alcohol consumption falls.

(a) *Alcoholic Tremulousness:* 'The shakes' may be of any severity from an inner feeling of the 'jitters' to severe agitation. Tremors of the hands and facial muscles are prominent.

(b) *Delirium Tremens:* This is an acute brain syndrome. There is a clouding of consciousness, extreme fear, restlessness, visual hallucinations and autonomic overactivity. The clinical picture characteristically fluctuates in severity, and subsides within 3-5 days. Generalized epileptic seizures often occur in the first 48 hours of the attack.

(5) *Alcoholic Hallucinosis*

In this uncommon syndrome auditory hallucinations occur; characteristically the patient hears voices talking about him. There is no clouding of consciousness. It is often difficult to differentiate this syndrome from schizophrenia. Some of the patients are in fact schizophrenics who are also alcoholics.

(6) *Chronic Brain Syndrome*

The main clinical features are those of other dementing illnesses (chapter 15).

The two following brain syndromes are seen in alcoholics and are associated with thiamine deficiency. Both can be caused by conditions other than alcoholism, e.g., Wernicke's can be caused by severe vomiting; Korsakoff's state by neoplasms or head injury.

(a) *Wernicke's Encephalopathy:* This is a rare condition. Pathologically there is a necrosis spread through the paraventricular regions of the thalamus and hypothalamus down the periaquaductal area to the floor of the 4th ventricle. The patient may seem alert, but he is disorientated and has memory impairment for recent events. Nystagmus should be present to make the diagnosis a 6th nerve palsy (with diplopia) may also be found. There may be a polyneuropathy. Thiamine is the essential medical treatment. The condition can be fatal, resolve completely, or proceed to:

(b) *Korsakoff's Syndrome:* This is an amnesic confabulatory syndrome in which peripheral neuritis may or may not be present. Memory for recent events is grossly impaired. Confabulation in varying degrees may be present. Response to treatment is usually incomplete.

PHYSICAL DISTURBANCES

These include fractures, head injuries (subdural haematoma), cirrhosis of the liver, peripheral neuritis, tuberculosis, hypoglycaemia, gastritis, cardiomyopathy and myopathy.

These will not be described here but each alcoholic patient must be examined carefully to see if any of these conditions are present.

SOCIAL DISTURBANCES

These include debts, broken marriages, lost jobs, motor accidents, crimes of violence and suicide. The effects within the family are profound and can only be fully appreciated when a patient's wife and children are seen.

DIAGNOSIS

It is essential to obtain an independent history of the patient's alcohol consumption. No reliance whatsoever can be attached to the patient's statements in this regard.

Information about the patient's behaviour at work and at home must be obtained from independent sources and a complete physical, psychiatric and social profile made.

PREVENTION AND TREATMENT

Prevention is the ideal, by general social measures and by detecting alcoholics before complications occur. Most alcoholics maintain their right to drink as and when they please, and are unable to face life without alcohol. If the alcoholic continues to refuse help, a crisis may have to be precipitated, e.g. his job could be suspended, and forced entry to hospital may have to be considered.

Treatment of alcoholism is a long process of re-education and rehabilitation.

The family doctor, psychiatrist, physician, surgeon, social worker, the church, employment officer, Alcoholics Anonymous, may all be involved at some stage of the treatment. Special centres are available in most cities where a team approach is used. It is best if one friendly but firm doctor can be responsible for the care of the patient, and he must be prepared for therapeutic failures. Repeated failures are the rule; only from these can the patient learn the reasons that underlie his drinking.

Once the patient has agreed to be helped, he should be admitted to a hospital or nursing home for several weeks and alcohol completely withdrawn. At this stage withdrawal symptoms can be controlled with tranquillizing drugs, e.g. diazepam (Valium) 10 mg. q.d.s., chlorpromazine (Largactil) 100-200 mg. q.d.s. Adequate food, vitamins and full supportive care (chapter 9) is given at this time.

Disulfiram (Antabuse) is a useful drug in selected cases (side effects include drowsiness, cardiovascular collapse, dermatitis, liver damage and peripheral neuritis. This drug is taken daily, the tablet usually being given by the wife. It should not be given without the patient's knowledge. Antabuse blocks an enzyme in the liver necessary to complete the breakdown of acetaldehyde which is an intermediate product in the metabolism of alcohol. The accumulation of acetaldehyde causes unpleasant symptoms—a sense of apprehension, facial flushing, precordial pain, nausea and vomiting. Usually the patient is allowed to experience such a reaction in hospital so that he can be aware of the consequences of taking alcohol with Antabuse.

Alcoholics Anonymous (A.A.) is a group of people who themselves have been alcoholic and who aim to help other alcoholics by a social and spiritual approach. This group approach may be a very helpful one for the isolated alcoholic and the patient should attend his first meetings from hospital. Psychotherapeutic groups are also used in the treatment of alcoholism.

Treatment of physical complications (if possible) is important, and depressive symptoms need treatment. The family and employment problems should be helped as much as possible.

Treatment of the Families

It is now recognized that the wife is usually not an innocent victim of her husband's drinking. Often they are insecure women who react to their husband's behaviour with active or passive aggression towards the husband. Sometimes, too, when the husband does stop drinking, the wife becomes depressed. Children of alcoholics often present problems at school, and there may be antisocial behaviour. The effect of the alcoholic father can have life long effects on the personality of the children. The problems of the wife and children therefore need to be looked at in each case individually.

PROGNOSIS

With this general approach, in socially stable alcoholics, improvement in about 40% of patients can be expected. Relapses, particularly at times of stress, should be expected and handled by the doctor with understanding, encouragement and firmness.

DRUG DEPENDENCE

In addition to alcohol, dependence on tobacco, marijuana, barbiturates, amphetamines, bromides, morphine, pethidine, heroin and cocaine present important medical and social problems.

Barbiturate addicts are often middle-aged while amphetamine addicts are usually young adults.

Barbiturates are commonly taken for sleeplessness and anxiety, while amphetamines are taken for fatigue, obesity, depression and to counter the effect of barbiturates. Many individuals take several drugs.

Excessive intake of barbiturates (or other sedatives) leads to ataxia, falls, fits, periods of stupor and delirium. If the patient denies taking drugs and this is believed, these clinical features can be mistaken for a neurological disorder or for neurotic symptoms.

Excessive intake of amphetamines can lead to the development of a paranoid illness that can be indistinguishable from paranoid schizophrenia. Detection of amphetamine-like substances in the urine may be helpful diagnostically. The symptoms subside over the course of 7-10 days after the amphetamines are withdrawn.

The young adolescent patient who 'uses' marijuana, amphetamine, cocaine, lysergic acid and other hallucinogenic drugs is an increasing medical and social problem. Some of the patients who reach psychiatrists, are schizophrenics who need treatment for this condition.

Social problems develop from drug dependence, in particular, the forging of medical prescriptions to obtain supplies of the drugs.

Prevention is obviously important, and these drugs are frequently given too readily in too large quantities. Prescriptions should therefore only be given after due thought and for a definite purpose. Amphetamines are of no value in depressive illness.

Treatment involves complete withdrawal of the drugs, using phenothiazines or benzodiazopines to minimize withdrawal symptoms. Full supportive care and a close follow up is needed. However, relapses are common.

The strict control of morphine, heroin and cocaine made these problems uncommon. When they did occur the patient was often a member of the medical, dental, nursing or pharmaceutical profession. Now, however, these drugs are part of the 'drug scene'. Analgesic abuse can lead to chronic renal damage.

SUMMARY

Alcoholism is an important problem in most countries. It should be recognized as a definite illness; stages in its development are described. See Appendix 6 for The Michigan Alcoholism Screening Test.

Physical, psychiatric and social disturbances are all important and should be defined in each patient.

Principles of treatment are discussed; the doctor must expect and make use of repeated failures.

Treatment is a long process of re-education and rehabilitation.

Drug dependence on barbiturates and amphetamines are important problems, the symptoms and problems raised are briefly described.

REFERENCES

Drew, L. R. M., Moon, J. R., Buchanan, F. H., *Alcoholism: a handbook*. (Heinemann, 1974). An Australian monograph that emphasizes the family and community aspects of alcoholism.

Kessell, N. and Walton, H., *Alcoholism*. Pelican (Harmondsworth 1974). A concise account of the many problems of alcoholism.

18

SUICIDE AND ATTEMPTED SUICIDE

Suicide and attempted suicide are important psychiatric problems about which students should be informed. Suicidal attempts are among the commonest non-traumatic conditions seen at the Casualty Department, and each general hospital usually deals with more than one such patient a day. Suicide itself is about 10th in any list of causes of deaths.

SUICIDE

Australia, Britain and the United States are countries that have a recorded suicide rate of between 10 and 14 per 100,000 of population. (In Australia fatal car accidents are about twice as frequent as recorded deaths from suicide). Some countries (Japan, East and West Germany) have a suicide rate of over 20 per 100,000, while other countries (Ireland and Spain) have a low suicide rate of 2-6 per 100,000. These differences between countries become important when one thinks about the general causes of suicide. It is relevant to note that if there have not been any great social changes the suicide rate of a country stays remarkably constant. It is important to realize that the *recorded* death rate from suicide is not the same as the *actual* death rate from suicide. Some authorities have indeed considered that the number of suicides recorded is no more than half those that actually occur. Suicide is an unpopular verdict in the coroner's court and relatives are rightly given the benefit of any doubt. In studies of suicide it is found that:

In all countries the suicide rate for men is greater than for women, the ratio being 2-3 men for 1 woman.

In all countries the average age for suicide is in the late fifties.

Certain other associations are also important:

Religion

Suicide rates among Roman Catholics, Jews and Moslems are usually below the average. Ireland, Spain and Italy have very low suicide rates, but other Roman Catholic countries—France, Austria and Hungary—have high rates.

Social Class

The suicide rate is highest in people engaged in professional and managerial occupations, followed by businessmen and executives. Doctors (and dentists) have a suicide rate one and a half times that of other males in Social Class 1. One in every 50 male doctors will die from suicide. Doctors' wives also have a high suicide rate. Under-graduates have a suicide rate significantly higher than that of the 17-24 years old group as a whole. Certain occupations have a low suicide rate, e.g., clergymen, railwaymen and coal-miners.

Loneliness

People who live alone have a high suicide rate (27% of suicides in London were living alone). Widowers have 5 times the normal suicide rate, while widows and divorced women have 3 times the normal rate. Divorced men between the ages of 61 and 70 have the highest suicide rate of all.

It has been found that in London and Chicago, the suicide rates were highest in those areas of the city where there are many hotels and lodging houses, while the suburban family areas have a low rate.

Seasonal Fluctuation

Suicide is more common in spring and early summer than in autumn and winter, but an adequate explanation for this phenomenon has still to be found.

Psychiatric Illness

Depressive illness is the psychiatric illness with the highest suicidal risk. In assessing the risk of suicide in a depressed patient it is import-ant to ask each depressed patient, 'Have you felt that life is not worth living?' Most depressed patients have experienced this and will welcome the opportunity to talk about it; one can then ask how bad the feeling gets and how they have controlled it (see chapter 12). Patients with *schizophrenia* sometimes commit suicide, usually in the early stages of the illness. Patients with *personality abnormalities* are among the other big group of psychiatric patients who commit suicide. Dependence on drugs or alcohol is often a factor here, as are the mood changes to which these personalities are prone.

Those factors associated with a high suicide and those with a low suicide rate are shown in Table 1.

Method of Suicide

Drug overdose is the commonest method of suicide. Other common methods include shooting, coal gas, hanging and jumping from high places. Some motor accidents are suicides.

Warning of Suicidal Attempt

60-75% of people who commit suicide have expressed the intention of committing suicide usually on several occasions. Despite this the act is a shock and surprise for relatives. 'People who threaten suicide do not carry it out' is an old medical adage completely without foundation. The opposite is in fact the truth.

Table 1

Factors associated with a high suicide rate	Factors associated with a low suicide rate
	Wars and revolutions
Economic crises	Favourable economic circumstances
Residence in large cities	Residence in country
Employment in industry	Rural occupations
Immigrants	
Certain occupations (e.g. businessmen, doctors, dentists, lawyers, students)	Certain occupations (e.g. clergymen, railwaymen, miners)
Protestant faith	Roman Catholic faith
Living alone	Living with family
Increasing age	Youth
Widowhood	
	Married state
Divorced state	
Childlessness	Large number of children
Psychiatric illness	
Alcoholism	

Prevention

The recognition of depressive illness and its treatment is the most important means of preventing suicides. Once recognized, certain clinical features are usually considered to indicate a high risk of suicide and these are detailed in chapter 12.

Studies of suicide have shown that in one group of patients (usually men) there is no past history of psychiatric illness, and the patients have recently developed severe depressive symptoms. The other group of patients (usually women) have a past history of psychiatric illness and may have made a previous suicidal attempt.

SUICIDAL ATTEMPTS

As has been stated suicidal attempts are much more frequent than suicide. Studying the facts of suicide and attempted suicide we see that there are some very striking differences:

(1) *Suicidal attempts* are much more frequent in women than men. *Suicide* is more frequent in men.

(2) The common age range for *suicidal attempts* is 15-30; that for *suicide* is 55+.

(3) Follow up of patients who have made *suicidal attempts* shows that as a rule *they do not die from suicide*. Repeated suicidal attempts are not unusual but only 1% of patients who have made them commit suicide in each year of such a follow up study.

These sorts of studies have shown that those people who *commit suicide* and those who *attempt suicide* are two different, though over-lapping, populations. The term 'suicide attempt' is in fact an inappropriate one, as it is often clear clinically that suicide is not in fact attempted and the term 'self poisoning' has been suggested as a more appropriate alternative, although this term also has limitations.

The typical clinical associations of a *suicide attempt* are a girl of 16-18 who after a succession of family rows about her boy friend, takes a small number of sleeping pills immediately after such an argument, then gets frightened and tells her parents what she has done. It is often done in a mood of 'I don't care if I live or die', and the attempt is in some ways a gamble, the outcome of which depends on various incidental factors. Aggression towards others is a motive easily seen in these patients. What is important in the suicidal attempt is the effect it has on the immediate family group. The incident mobilizes profound anxiety from all the people involved. Suicidal attempts are therefore best considered *as an appeal to the environment*. The *social implications* of the act are of great importance and should be studied in every case. In hospital it is of great value to find out who visits the patient and what happens during these visits. This information often gives important clues in managing the patient.

In women, both *suicides* and *suicidal attempts* are more frequent in the premenstrual phase of the menstrual cycle. In one study of 70 female suicides, 7 were pregnant, 35 were menstruating and 1 was in the puerperium. Of the women under 45 who committed suicide, two-thirds were either menstruating or in the premenstrual phase of the cycle.

General management of a patient admitted to hospital after a 'suicide attempt'

The care of the unconscious patient is an important skill, details of which should be obtained from textbooks of medicine. A full history must be obtained from relatives (or neighbours if the patient lives alone), so that the events leading to the suicidal attempt can be established. The patient when conscious and co-operative must of course be given adequate time to tell her own story. Two usual clinical situations are found:

(1) that there is a history of definite persistent depressive symptoms and the incident was really unsuccessful, a failed suicide.

(2) that the suicidal attempt was the consequence of a reaction to some interpersonal difficulties.

In the former case, appropriate anti-depressive treatment is indicated, and the patient should have improved considerably before being discharged from hospital.

In the latter case, the changing relationships with parents or boy friend that occur because of the suicidal attempt are important. Usually after a few days the situation that led to the attempt is resolved and the patient can leave hospital to attend later for outpatient care.

If the situation does not resolve, social and psychiatric treatment is needed, privately or at an outpatient or day hospital level. These patients usually have persistent neurotic or personality problems and may already have made several suicidal attempts. As has been mentioned the actual risk of suicide in these patients is small, but they are best treated by a psychiatrist.

SUMMARY

Suicide and attempted suicide are important problems; the differences between them are emphasized.

Suicide usually occurs in elderly men, suicidal attempts in young women.

Suicides are usually associated with depressive illness; methods of assessing the suicidal risk in a depressed patient are emphasized.

Suicidal attempts usually result from the reaction of a neurotic personality with interpersonal problems.

REFERENCES

Stengel, E., *Suicide and Attempted Suicide*. Pelican (Harmondsworth, 1973). A popular account by an expert in this field.

Farmer, R. and Hirsch, S. (eds), *The Suicide Syndrome*. Croom Helm (London, 1980). A recent symposium on these topics.

19

SCHIZOPHRENIA

The name schizophrenia was given by Bleuler in 1911 to *a group of grave and common psychiatric illnesses characterized by a special type of thought disorder and disturbances in the volitional and emotional life of the patient.*

In all countries patients with chronic schizophrenia occupy about half of all hospital beds. The clinical problems of schizophrenia for the non-psychiatrist are essentially diagnosis in early cases, and the management of patients when they are discharged from hospitals.

The term schizophrenia probably includes a number of different illnesses with common symptoms. It is useful, clinically, to regard the concept of schizophrenia today in the same light as the old concept of Bright's disease. Bright's disease was a term given to patients with albuminuria, hypertension and oedema. It is now known that a number of different pathological lesions account for this syndrome. Research into schizophrenia may well enable a similar 'breakdown' of the syndrome to occur.

Further it has to be appreciated that classical schizophrenic symptoms can occur in the course of other illnesses, e.g., acute brain syndromes (chapter 15), cerebral tumours, temporal lobe epilepsy. Amphetamines taken in large doses by addicts can produce a schizophrenic-like syndrome.

AETIOLOGY

The causes of schizophrenia are not fully known. As a working hypothesis the illness can be considered to be the result of some endogenous toxic process in an individual predisposed to succumb because of hereditary factors.

These hereditary factors have been shown in studies of the incidence of schizophrenia in identical and non-identical twins. If one twin has schizophrenia and he is one of a dizygotic pair, the other twin is likely to have a similar illness in about 15% of cases. If he is one of a monozygotic pair the chance of the other twin having schizophrenia is about 40%. Recent studies of children from a schizophrenic parent, but adopted at birth by other families have attempted to sort out the 'nature'/'nurture' argument in the aetiology of schizophenia. Evidence to support the importance of a genetic background to schizophrenia has been found.

Schizophrenia occurs in all races, in all cultures and the incidence rate is roughly the same—it affects 0·85% of the population. Parents of schizophrenics are likely to have a history of a similar illness in about 10% of cases.

Mode of Inheritance of Genetic Predisposition

This is not known, but a single partially dominant gene, or a recessive inheritance with a partial penetrance are the two main suggestions.

Premorbid Personality

About half the patients who develop schizophrenia have an apparently normal personality before the onset of their illness. Others show 'schizoid' traits, i.e. solitariness, shyness, callousness and eccentricity.

Sex and the Age of Onset

75% of patients develop symptoms between the ages of 15-25 years. Schizophrenia with paranoid symptoms often develops after the age of 40. There is also a schizophrenic syndrome in childhood.

Females are affected slightly more than males.

Research into Aetiology

Research into schizophrenia has grown enormously in the past 10 years. This has included social and epidemiological studies, psychodynamic approaches to schizophrenia and psychological studies of thought disorder and perceptual abnormalities. The largest group of researches have been devoted to biochemical investigations; but the difficulties in investigating biochemical mechanisms in the brain are great. Certain so called 'hallucinogenic' drugs can produce abnormalities in normal subjects that are similar to those seen in schizophrenia. These observations have been the foundation for many of the biochemical theories of schizophrenia.

One such drug is *mescaline* which has a chemical structure similar to adrenaline. One theory of schizophrenia relates the illness to faulty metabolism of adrenaline.

Another hallucinogenic drug, *lysergic acid diethylamide* (L.S.D.), antagonizes the action of serotonin on smooth muscle. One theory of schizophrenia relates the illness to abnormalities in brain serotonin.

It is known that methylation of serotonin, derivatives of tryptamine and adrenaline can produce hallucinogenic compounds. It has therefore been suggested that some disorder in methylation may be associated with schizophrenia.

All the drugs that relieve schizophrenic symptoms, e.g. the phenothiazines and butyrephenones, produce an unwanted effect—extrapyramidal symptoms. These and the therapeutic effects are thought to be dependent upon central dopamine receptor blockade. This is an important biochemical hypothesis for studies in schizophrenia.

Amphetamine, the substance that can produce a clinical picture most like schizophrenia, produces its effects in the brain via dopamine receptors.

PRECIPITATING FACTORS

Physical Precipitation

Schizophrenic illness can develop after childbirth, surgical operations and physical illness.

Psychological Precipitation

Care is needed in assessing this because of the usual insidious onset of the illness. Early symptoms, e.g. failure to concentrate can produce poor examination results, which can then be blamed as a precipitating factor. Similarly, emotional changes produced by the illness can cause disturbances in interpersonal relationships with fiancé or parents that can then be incriminated as a precipitating cause.

Some popular theories of causation have regarded schizophrenia as an understandable reaction to deviances in the patient's family. In its simplest form, the patient who becomes schizophrenic is subjected to a series of conflicting communications which he cannot resolve. Some psychiatrists have extended this concept and regard schizophrenia as a healthy reaction to the constraints of family and society! Such theories have become popular in non medical circles. Studies of communications in families with a schizophrenic member have in fact produced no evidence to support theories of family deviance and schizophrenia. There are no sound reasons to put the onus of the schizophrenic's illness on his immediate family; *there is no evidence for it and it is poor clinical practice.*

ONSET

In most instances the illness is of gradual onset, and the actual course of the illness can only be judged by a full history obtained from all relevant sources. Sometimes the symptoms develop acutely over the course of a few weeks.

CLINICAL FEATURES

The main abnormalities can be described under the following headings:

Disorder of Thinking

Normal thinking is orderly and clear—*schizophrenic thinking is disorderly and woolly.* Patients give vague answers to questions. At the end of a long interview one often feels that no definite information or impression of the patient is gained. In schizophrenia, ideas may not be associated in a logical fashion, but by internal and external stimuli which the schizophrenic cannot ignore. Irrelevant ideas and phantasies therefore get involved in their thinking. Sometimes difficulty in thinking is shown only in response to proverbs—when patients give 'concrete' answers. However, such answers are not necessarily diagnostic of schizophrenia, as patients of low intelligence also give 'concrete' answers.

Disorder of Emotions

There is a progressive emotional blunting so that 'laughter holds no mirth and tears no sorrow'. Sometimes the patient may be speaking of sad things and laugh or vice versa. This splitting of the emotions from the appropriate thoughts is called incongruity of affect. Schizophrenic emotional changes can produce in the doctor the feeling that there is a pane of glass between the patient and himself—there is no communication of affect. With experience this is a valuable clinical observation.

Disorder of Volition

There is a progressive blunting of will power. Patients find it more and more difficult to take an interest in things. They tend to stay in bed late and get progressively more inactive, *they retreat into their inner world (autism)* which itself is disrupted, particularly by—

Hallucinations

These are important phenomena in schizophrenia. They occur in clear consciousness (i.e. patient is not disorientated) and are usually auditory. Somatic hallucinations are not uncommon but visual ones are rare.

Kraepelin gave a masterly description of auditory hallucinations—'The hallucinations of hearing begin as simple noises, rustling, banging, singing in the ears, music, ringing, whistling. There then develops, gradually or suddenly a hearing of voices. Sometimes as a whisper, sometimes loud or like a telephone. Sometimes a chorus, sometimes the voices seem to be thoughts with words. They are often referred to a particular ear and sometimes they seem to come from inside the body. Usually however, the voices come from the external world. The voices usually say unpleasant or disturbing things, but sometimes the voices are "good". Commonly the patient's own thoughts appear to be spoken out "loud".'

While the neurophysiological basis of these hallucinations is not known psychopathological explanations of the *content* of the hallucinations are often valuable, e.g., the young male schizophrenic with voices concerned with his homosexual problems.

Delusional Ideas

Many 'secondary' delusional ideas develop as an explanation for other symptoms, e.g., hallucinations or emotional changes. A patient with auditory hallucinations 'explained' these as being due to a radio transmitter which the doctors had put into his arm at the time of an operation for a compound fracture of the humerus.

A patient who feels different may recognize this and 'explain' this by believing someone is drugging him.

Some delusional ideas seem to develop de novo—when they are called primary delusions.

Mental Functions not Altered

It is important to recognize that in schizophrenia there are usually no disturbances of consciousness, memory or intelligence—as in the organic psychiatric disorders.

Usual Clinical Presentation

Parents may bring an adolescent boy to their family doctor because *gradually* he has become more solitary, and his school work has deteriorated. He may be taking no interest in his appearance, not going out with friends and being disobedient at home. Some recent episode may have made the parents realize that their child is ill. Sometimes this episode is some gross social blunder or the boy may have accused his parents of poisoning him.

On examination, the patient may seem apathetic and indifferent and unable to account for his parents' concern. He may be quite unable to realize that he has changed. This sort of clinical problem at once raises the possibility of schizophrenia and the patient should be referred to a psychiatrist in order to confirm the diagnosis and advise treatment. Definite diagnosis and management of this serious illness is a problem for the psychiatrist. Often these patients will be admitted to hospital for 4-6 weeks for assessment and treatment and then sent home, when the family doctor must be aware of the treatment programme—essential to which is usually the long term administration of phenothiazine drugs.

DIFFERENTIAL DIAGNOSIS

This again is essentially a problem for psychiatrists, and need not be entered into here. If a patient seems to have one or other of the clinical features described, he should be referred for expert opinion. Several interviews with the patient and relatives may be necessary before a firm diagnosis can be made. The terms 'early' or 'latent' or 'incipient' or 'borderline' schizophrenia should be avoided.

The diagnosis is a clinical one which should be made on a detailed study of a full history from independent sources and observation of the patient. *There are no tests, physical or psychological, that can establish the diagnosis for the clinician.*

CLINICAL TYPES

As has been mentioned schizophrenia probably includes a number of different entities. Certain clinical types can be recognized, but an individual patient may show mainly hebephrenic features at one time and paranoid features at another.

Simple Type

Here there is an insidious onset; there are no florid features, and the patients may be apathetic drifters who never see a doctor.

Hebephrenic Type

This begins in adolescence with thought disorder and hallucinations and is the usual type of schizophrenia.

Catatonic Type

Here disorders of movement from stupor to overactivity are the main findings. This is an unusual type of schizophrenia.

Paranoid Type

Delusions and hallucinations are the prominent phenomena. Thought disorder, emotional and volitional disorders are less obvious. These patients are often over 40.

COURSE OF THE ILLNESS

The illness usually runs a chronic course and is not a fatal one except for the risk of suicide. *Before modern treatments* the outcome was usually stated as:

25% end with severe deterioration
25% end with marked personality deterioration
25% end with mild personality deterioration
25% recover completely.

Often there are a series of 'attacks' with the personality deterioration being more marked after each attack.

PROGNOSIS

Age

The younger the patient is when the illness starts the worse is the prognosis.

Onset

An acute onset is a favourable sign.

Premorbid Personality

A normal premorbid personality is a good prognostic feature.

Precipitating Cause

The presence of a definite precipitating cause is a good sign (e.g. childbirth).

Pyknic Body Build

(i.e. heavily built—John Bull physique) may be associated with relatively benign symptoms.

The insidious onset of classical symptoms with no apparent cause in an adolescent with schizoid personality features are clinical associations with a bad prognosis.

PREVENTION AND TREATMENT

Prevention

No preventative measures are at present possible. Children with one schizophrenic parent have about a 10% chance of developing the illness. Two schizophrenics not infrequently marry and here the risk is considerably more.

Treatment

Treatment of an illness like schizophrenia which usually runs a chronic course is a complex matter that involves social, psychological and physical aspects in the whole therapeutic programme.

Treatment discussed here will be on the patient admitted to hospital for the first time with a schizophrenic illness and his management thereafter. The management of the chronic patient will not be discussed in any detail.

The general aim should be to admit schizophrenic patients with an acute illness to hospital for short periods; to initiate active physical treatments and to make any social adjustments necessary. The patients should then return to their family and job and continue with medication and supportive care indefinitely. This supportive care may well be shared by the G.P. and the psychiatrist at a psychiatric out-patient clinic or in private practice.

In hospital, the treatment of the illness usually involves treatment with tranquillizing drugs and sometimes a short course of E.C.T. along with general social rehabilitative measures. E.C.T. is usually given 2 or 3 times a week for 6-8 treatments—its effect on schizophrenic illness is often to diminish the intensity of delusional and hallucinatory activity. These symptoms will return however unless medication with tranquillizing drugs is also commenced. [E.C.T. may be the only treatment necessary in the rare catatonic form of schizophrenia and in schizophrenia precipitated by childbirth and operations.]

The tranquillizing drugs will be discussed in chapter 20. Usually long term treatment with one of the piperazine phenothiazines e.g. trifluoperazine (Stelazine) is the treatment of choice. The use of these phenothiazine drugs has completely altered the outlook for patients with schizophrenic illness. Medication must be continued once the patient leaves hospital for *several years* in the majority of cases. Barbiturates are of no permanent value in treating schizophrenic symptoms; anti-depressant drugs are sometimes helpful in treating depressive symptoms if they develop in a particular patient.

For some patients who will not take medication regularly the use of long acting preparations given every 2 or 3 weeks by intramuscular injection (e.g. fluphenazine decanoate (Modecate)) has been an important recent advance in the treatment of schizophrenic patients.

Supportive Care

This is of the utmost importance in the care of schizophrenic patients and their families. The social and personal problems that these patients develop can often be minimized by regular supportive care from one interested doctor. He must be prepared to look after these young patients who usually have considerable problems in their relationships with other people. The illness may develop at a time when engagement and marriage problems are to the fore, and supportive care through these times, as well as any pregnancies, needs considerable clinical skill. *Psychotherapy proper is contra-indicated for these patients.*

Unfortunately, despite the best possible care, relapses occur. Sometimes this is associated with the patient stopping the tranquillizing drugs. Further hospital admissions may be necessary, but these should be as brief as possible. It is not known how many schizophrenic patients today will need long term hospital admission in spite of modern treatment as tranquillizing drugs were only introduced in 1953.

The treatment of *chronic schizophrenia* is a more complex problem. Social and rehabilitative measures are of great importance, while tranquillizing drugs are also of value. It has been found that schizophrenic patients discharged from hospital often do best at a hostel or in lodgings, rather than living at home with their parents. Disruptive emotional problems are more likely to occur at home and the family doctor may have to help the parents accept this. Work is of the greatest importance in the rehabilitation of the chronic schizophrenic. Sheltered workshops are available in some centres, but work in the community no matter how menial or monotonous the job may appear to the parents, must be actively encouraged. Regular psychiatric attention will be needed for these chronic patients in order to assess all aspects of the patient's progress.

SUMMARY

The term 'schizophrenia' is used to describe a group of illnesses of essentially unknown origin.

The main symptoms are associated with disorders of thinking, volition and emotions, as well as auditory hallucinations and delusional ideas.

Treatment with phenothiazine drugs has transformed the outlook for schizophrenic patients.

Long stay hospital admission is now the exception rather than the rule.

The importance of supportive treatment is emphasized.

REFERENCE

Bleuler, E., *Dementia Praecox or the Group of Schizophrenics*. Allen & Unwin (London, 1949). The classical monograph on this group of illnesses.

20

TRANQUILLIZING DRUGS
AND HYPNOTICS

The drug treatment of psychiatric symptoms is an important aspect of present day psychiatric practice. It is no exaggeration to say that these drugs have completely revolutionized treatment in psychiatry. It is important that students should be aware of certain principles that will guide them in this expanding field of practical psychiatry, and know how to use a small number of the compounds available.

Drugs which influence the 'higher functions' of the brain are known collectively as *psychotropic* drugs. This general term includes sedatives, stimulants, anti-depressants, hallucinogenic and tranquillizing drugs. This last term was originally applied to chlorpromazine and reserpine because of their ability to quieten a disturbed patient, without the sedative qualities of the barbiturates. In the group of tranquillizers there are now a very large number of drugs which possess differing types of pharmacological activity.

Most of the highly potent clinically effective tranquillizers are *phenothiazines*. The basic structure of the phenothiazine molecule is shown in Figure 2.

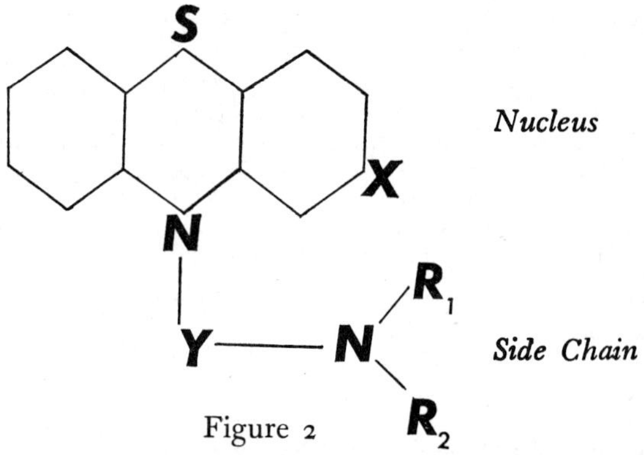

Figure 2

Phenothiazines can be divided into three groups by the structure of their side chains:

(1) One has *methyl* groups at R_1 and R_2, and is the *dimethyl group* (e.g., chlorpromazine, promazine).

(2) Another group of more potent compounds, has a piperazine ring at R_1 or R_2 and is the *piperazine group* (e.g., trifluoperazine, perphenazine).

(3) Another group has a *piperidine* nucleus in the side chain (e.g., thioridazine). This group produces fewer side effects but is of variable potency.

The nature of X in the nucleus also determines potency. Chlorpromazine has a Cl, while trifluoperazine has a CF_3 grouping at X. The more potent piperazine phenothiazines seem to alert patients and readily produce extrapyramidal side effects, while the dimethyl phenothiazines tend to produce sedation and side effects of dermatitis, hypotension and jaundice. The piperidine group, as has been mentioned, has fewer side effects.

Other drugs which are tranquillizers include haloperidol (Serenace), chemically a butyrophenone; and members of a large group of muscle relaxing drugs used in patients with relatively mild symptoms, the benzodiazepines, e.g. diazepam (Valium). This last drug is also valuable for patients with an acute brain syndrome as it can be given systemically. In addition, it has few side effects and overdose is not lethal.

COMMONLY USED TRANQUILLIZING DRUGS

Name	Trade Name (*Tablet size; mg.*)	Usual Adult Dose Range (*mg./day*)	Important Side Effects
1. PHENOTHIAZINES			
Chlor-promazine	Largactil Thorazine (10,25,50,100)	75—1,000	Drowsiness, jaundice, fits, photosensitization, hypotension
Trifluo-perazine	Stelazine (1,2,5,10)	6—60	Extrapyramidal syndrome
Perphenazine	Trilafon (2,4,8,16)	6—64	Extrapyramidal syndrome
Thioridazine	Melleril (10,25,50,100)	75—600	Few at usual dosage; impotence
2. BUTYROPHENONES			
Haloperidol	Serenace (0·5, 1·5)	3—20	Extrapyramidal syndrome
Pimozide	Orap (2)	2—10	Extrapyramidal syndrome
3. MILDER 'MUSCLE RELAXANT' TRANQUILLIZERS			
Diazepam	Valium (2,5,10)	6—30	Ataxia, drowsiness, dependence
Lorazepam	Ativan (1, 2.5)	2—10	Ataxia, drowsiness, dependence
Oxazepam	Adumbran Serepax (10,15,30)	10—30	Ataxia, drowsiness, dependence

It is not necessary to list the very large number of tranquillizers that are currently available. Attention is directed to a small number of drugs about which dosage and side effects should be known.

Mode of Action

The mode of action of these drugs in psychiatric illness is still not clearly known. The drugs certainly have effects on the hypothalamus and brain stem reticular formation, but perhaps it is their central action that is most important. Their effect in blocking dopamine receptors is probably of particular importance.

Specific benzodiazepine receptor sites have recently been found in the C.N.S.

SIDE EFFECTS AND THEIR MANAGEMENT

Skin Eruptions

Allergic reactions (including urticaria, macular and acne-like eruptions) and photosensitivity. These are frequent with the dimethyl group of phenothiazines. The drug should be stopped and another phenothiazine prescribed (e.g. thioridazine). Skin pigmentation (and in the lens and cornea) have been reported with large doses of chlorpromazine given for several years.

Jaundice

This is of obstructive type, occurring in the first month or two of treatment. Fatalities are rare. Seen mainly with chlorpromazine.

Hypotension

Postural hypotensive symptoms are seen with the dimethyl group in the first few weeks of treatment.

Drowsiness

This is a common symptom in first few weeks of treatment with the dimethyl group.

Autonomic and other Symptoms

These are frequent with all the main tranquillizers but are usually not complained of after the first few weeks of treatment. Complaints include dry mouth, constipation, blurred vision, weight gain, oedema, vivid dreams, lactation, menstrual changes.

Blood Dyscrasias

Agranulocytosis is a rare complication of treatment with tranquillizing drugs.

Extrapyramidal Syndrome

The extrapyramidal syndrome is an important, frequent, reversible side effect of treatment with potent tranquillizers. It is made up of the following components:

(1) *Akathisia:* This is a motor restlessness—an inability to sit still—an inner disquiet or jitters. It is a very frequent complaint in the first few days of treatment with piperazine phenothiazines and haloperidol. It does not respond to anti-parkinsonian drugs but usually settles down over the course of a week or two. If treatment is needed temporarily, then chlorpromazine 50 mg. t.d.s. or diazepam 5 mg. t.d.s. is helpful.

(2) *Parkinsonism:* Characterized by gait and postural abnormalities—rigidity, tremor and salivation. Note particularly facial signs and non-swinging of arms as patient walks.

(3) *Dystonias:* These include perioral spasms, torticollis, mandibular tics, occulogyric crises and hyperextension of the neck. These symptoms occur usually when I.M. phenothiazines or haloperidol are given without anti-parkinsonian drugs. I.V. Cogentin relieves symptoms immediately. These effects can occur if these drugs are given in large doses by mouth, particularly in children, adolescents and the elderly.

(4) *Akinesia:* Weakness of muscles may be a temporary symptom occurring in the first few weeks of treatment.

(5) *Tardive Dyskinesia:* The syndrome can occur in patients on long-term treatment with major tranquillizers, or may occur some time after drug treatment has been stopped (hence the name 'tardive'). It tends to occur in more elderly patients, especially women. The symptoms are persistent and are rhythmical involuntary movements of the tongue, face, mouth and jaw. Anti-parkinsonian agents do not relieve the symptoms. The dosage and continuance of the major tranquillizer needs to be reviewed.

These extrapyramidal symptoms are reversed by stopping the tranquillizer or adding anti-parkinsonian drugs but *they can be prevented.*

Prevention

(a) by using thioridazine that does not usually produce this syndrome.

(b) by increasing dosage of drugs slowly and perhaps giving them in one dose per day (at bedtime).

(c) by giving anti-parkinsonian drugs with the tranquillizer, e.g. benztropine (Cogentin) 2 mg. b.d., orphenadrine (Disipal) 50 mg. t.d.s. It is wise to do this when any tranquillizer is given by injection; also with haloperidol given orally; when the piperazine group are given in large doses for long periods of time (e.g. over 20 mg. Stelazine per day). Note that children and elderly people are particularly liable to develop these side effects.

Name	Trade Name (*Tablet size in mg.*)	Usual Adult Dose Range (*mg./day*)
Orphenadrine	Disipal (50)	50—300
Benztropine	Cogentin (2)	0·5—6
Benzhexol	Artane, Pipanol (2)	6—10
Procyclidine	Kemadrin (5)	2·5—10

*These drugs can occasionally produce a confusional state. Some, e.g. benztropine, are available for I.M. and I.V. injections. All these drugs seem equally effective in preventing or treating drug-induced parkinsonism.

Side Effects with E.C.T. and other Drugs

In the usual dosage, all these drugs can be given with E.C.T. and the accompanying anaesthesia. Fatalities were originally reported with very large doses of chlorpromazine (over 1000 mg. per day). *Monoamine oxidase inhibitors* can potentiate the action of these drugs and care is needed in prescribing both sets of drugs together.

All these compounds are used in varying doses in different clinical settings. They are used essentially for patients who show clinical features of *agitation, anxiety, hallucinations* or *disorientation*.

The actual clinical syndromes for which they are used include:

(1) the acute brain syndrome from any cause (e.g. alcohol).

(2) the chronic brain syndrome from any cause (e.g. senile dementia).

(3) schizophrenia either with acute or chronic symptoms.

(4) manic patients.

(5) anxious patients.

(6) agitated patients (e.g. severe depression or obsessional neurosis).

(7) a number of other '*various*' conditions, e.g. chorea, torticollis, tics, psychosomatic conditions, behavioural disorders in children, painful conditions, treatment of drug dependence, vomiting, etc.

To simplify the wide range of clinical usage, the drug treatment (*which is only part of the whole treatment*), is described in the following 'typical' examples.

(1) A heavily built man of 40 develops symptoms of the acute brain syndrome soon after an operation for acute appendicitis. He is known to drink beer regularly in large quantities. I.V. diazepam 10-20 mg. to be repeated as needed for 12 hours. Then oral diazepam 10 mg. q.d.s. given for another 3 days. In addition large doses of multivitamin preparation are given by injection for 3 days.

(2) An elderly man has memory loss, is restless and 'difficult' at night. 100 mg. chlorpromazine or thioridazine nocte. If a similar patient also has deteriorating social habits in the day, regular medication—thioridazine 50 mg. t.d.s. may be helpful.

(3a) A young woman is admitted to hospital with unusual behaviour and auditory hallucinations. A diagnosis of schizophrenia is made. A course of 6 ECT is given and trifluoperazine (Stelazine) 20 mg. nocte given with Cogentin 2 mg. Later the trifluoperazine dosage may need to be increased to 40 mg. nocte and continued for at least 2 years as an out-patient.

(3b) A patient who has been diagnosed as schizophrenic many years ago is readmitted to hospital, withdrawn and apathetic. He is unreliable in taking tablets. Fluphenazine decanoate (Modecate) is given by intramuscular injection. 25 mg. as a starting dose, then 25-100 mg. each 2-4 weeks. In addition an anti-parkinsonian drug is given daily by mouth, e.g. Cogentin 2 mg.

(4) Very disturbed man with manic symptoms. Haloperidol (Serenace) 20 mg. i.v. stat., then 5 mg. i.v. 3-hourly, along with anti-parkinsonian drugs. Then when the patient quietens, give drugs by mouth, e.g. 10 mg. haloperidol + 2 mg. Cogentin b.d. Continue drugs for several weeks or months, then withdraw them gradually.

(5) The problems of treating anxiety with drugs is a complicated one, and drugs usually *play only a minor role in the total treatment*. These problems are discussed in chapter 10.

(6) A severely depressed, agitated man, starting treatment with E.C.T. is also given diazepam (Valium) 10 mg. t.d.s. for the first 10 to 14 days to ease the symptoms of agitation until the 'anti-depressant' treatment begins to be effective.

(7) A patient with a painful amputation stump is given chlorpromazine 100 mg. t.d.s. and codeine rather than more powerful analgesics.

It is again important to emphasize that while these drugs *sometimes completely* relieve symptoms, it is more usual for them to *greatly ease* the symptoms so that general nursing, social and psychiatric care can be carried out more effectively.

HYPNOTICS

Sleep disturbances are common complaints of psychiatric patients, but many insomniacs do not have psychiatric symptoms. Such disturbances are a cardinal feature of depression, mania and anxiety states. The more common clinical problem is the patient with particular problems at home or at work. It is important to take a full history from the patient, and to consider whether the symptoms of depression are present.

Before prescribing an hypnotic, it is important to recognize that once these are used regularly, then if stopped, sleep becomes disturbed because of withdrawal symptoms and convinces the patient that sleeping pills are essential.

As regards hypnotics, benzodiazepines such as nitrazepam (Mogadon), flurazepam (Dalmane) and diazepam (Valium) are effective and safe. Barbiturates are unsafe. New, short acting benzodiazepines have recently been introduced. They include lorazepam (Ativan), temazepam (Euhypnos, Normison), midazolam and triazolam. Because of their short action they may prove to be the hypnotics of choice.

SUMMARY

Tranquillizing drugs are described; most are phenothiazines. These drugs have completely altered psychiatric practice since their introduction in 1953. They are of great value in schizophrenia.

Their mode of action is still ill defined.

Some typical clinical examples are given of the use of these drugs.

A brief account of hypnotics is given.

Students are advised to learn how to use a few tranquillizing drugs properly.

REFERENCE

Sargant, W. and Slater, E., assisted by D. Kelly, *An Introduction to Physical Methods of Treatment in Psychiatry.* 5th ed., Livingstone (Edinburgh, 1972). The best account of this subject.

21

DRUG TRIALS AND PLACEBOS

The drug treatment of psychiatric illnesses is now an important aspect of the family doctor's work. It has already been mentioned that the assessment of the value of drugs in psychiatry is difficult, particularly in the neuroses and in depression. Because of this, it is important that a student should understand the basic principles of drug evaluation in psychiatric patients. Without this knowledge, he will be unable to examine critically statements from the drug companies when he is qualified.

As has been mentioned the practical value of these drugs has been enormous; they have helped transform psychiatric hospitals and have completely altered the outlook for many psychiatric patients. In addition, from a theoretical view point, the study of their mode of action should help unravel some of the unknowns of psychiatric illness, e.g. some drugs reduce the intensity of the auditory hallucinations of schizophrenic patients. If the mode of action of these drugs can be defined, then hypotheses about the causation of these hallucinations can be suggested and tested. This whole field of study is now known as *psychopharmacology*.

In order to assess the therapeutic value of a drug a *controlled trial* is essential. In such a trial, the drug is used in a particular dosage, for a specified length of time, in patients suffering from a particular disease or group of symptoms. The effects are compared with those produced either by an inert substance, or by an equivalent dose of a similar substance of known activity, given for the same length of time, in a similar group of patients (i.e. the control group). Before the trial starts, and throughout its course, measurements of change are made by observers who are unaware what treatment the patients are receiving (double blind technique). The results of the trial are finally assessed by appropriate statistical methods.

In psychiatric illness, certain problems present themselves:

(1) It has been emphasized that many of the 'labels' for diseases in psychiatry probably cover a number of distinct entities. We also have no objective criteria to establish the presence of these illnesses (e.g. there are no tests for schizophrenia or depressive illness). We have therefore to lay down operational definitions of the illnesses we are studying and try to ensure that different observers use these definitions in the same way.

(2) The actual trial must be conducted in a 'stable' environment; in theory, everything should be uniform except that one patient has the active drug and the control patient the inert substance. In practice,

there should be no changes in ward routine when drug trials are in progress. Trials in out-patients are difficult because of variable environmental factors, and also because the patients cannot be relied upon to take their tablets regularly and not to take other medication.

(3) The dose of active drugs and length of time they are to be taken for are decided before the trial starts. Different doses may give different results.

(4) Trials are of two sorts:

(a) where the patient himself is used as a control. Usually for one month the patient has one sort of treatment, for the next month another sort of treatment is given. This assumes that the clinical state of the patient would remain stationary over this length of time. This assumption is usually only valid in patients with chronic symptoms. This type of trial is called a *cross over trial.*

(b) where patients are *matched* and treatment allocated by random methods. Age, sex, intelligence, social class, length, form and severity of illness should all be carefully matched. Matching pairs of patients in psychiatry is a difficult problem because the fundamental causes of severe psychiatric illnesses are not known, e.g. if 'schizophrenia' has a number of different pathologies with common symptoms, matching by symptoms only may be erroneous.

(5) In assessing progress of patients, doctors and nurses must not know what treatment the particular patients are receiving—the so-called *blind trial.* In medicine, assessment of progress can be made by objective tests (e.g. E.S.R. or radiographic changes in pulmonary tuberculosis); this is not possible in psychiatry where standard rating scales of severity of symptoms are used. If carefully devised, and the assessors experienced and 'blind', these scales are valid and reliable measuring techniques.

(6) Results of the trial must be assessed by appropriate statistical methods, to determine whether the results obtained could have been obtained by chance.

A typical trial in psychiatry would be to compare a new anti-depressive compound with a standard drug (e.g. imipramine) in patients admitted to hospital with a primary depressive illness. Another frequent exercise is to compare two different tranquillizers in patients with chronic schizophrenia. Trials of drugs on anxious patients are also important.

Few of the reported drug trials meet all these requirements. In general, those that do have been carried out on hospitalized patients with severe psychiatric illnesses. Trials on outpatients or patients attending the family doctor with milder illnesses are usually open to methodological criticism, so that the value of drugs in these more numerous patients is extremely difficult to assess. Generalizations from the results of trials on severe hospitalized patients to patients in the community with milder symptoms may not be valid. Environmental and psychological factors are much more likely to affect the course of these milder illnesses; *hence the value of drugs in their treatment is probably over-rated.*

PLACEBOS

It has been known for many years that certain groups of symptoms —e.g. pains, seasickness, headaches, anxiety, depression symptoms can all be relieved with inert substances in about 30% of patients. The patent medicine industry depends upon this fact. The inert substance may be saline, lactose, chalk or substances in homeopathic doses. Collectively they are known as *placebos*.

Placebos can produce not only relief of symptoms but also side effects, e.g. dry mouth, nausea, headache, drowsiness, fatigue, palpitations, diarrhoea, constipation.

Certain factors are known to be associated with the 'potency' of placebos—the size, colour, taste and the route of administration are important. Who gives it and in what manner are also important.

However, using similar placebos given by the same doctor in the same manner, some patients respond to them, while others do not. Studies of these *placebo reactors* have shown that they are more sociable, more talkative, more appreciative of doctors and hospitals than other patients. Intelligence and sex are not important in this respect, but placebo reactors are more extraverted and show more neurotic trends than non-reactors.

Attention is now focused on the transactional nature of the doctor-patient relationship; in particular, the patient's faith in his doctor and the treatment given, and the doctor's confidence and belief in his mode of treatment. These are the main ingredients of many successful modes of treatment. In discussing placebo reaction, attention should be focused on these transactional processes, rather than the inert tablet used. These so-called *'nonspecific'* factors are of great therapeutic importance in medicine but are a problem when one is trying to separate out *'specific'* drug response in a treatment situation.

SUMMARY

The methodology of controlled drug trials in psychiatry is described, and the difficulties emphasized.

Such trials are essential to assess the value of drugs.

Nonspecific factors in drug treatment are briefly discussed.

REFERENCES

Witts, L. J. (ed.), *Medical Surveys and Clinical Trials.* Oxford University Press, 1964. A useful review of the problems of trials in medicine.

Beecher, H. K., *Measurement of Subjective Responses.* Oxford University Press (New York, 1959). This book has excellent chapters on pain and placebos.

22

THE PREMENSTRUAL SYNDROME—PSYCHIATRIC SYMPTOMS AND PREGNANCY—THE MENOPAUSE

THE PREMENSTRUAL SYNDROME

The premenstrual syndrome includes a wide variety of symptoms that occur regularly at the same phase of each menstrual cycle. These symptoms are common and frequently severe when they affect not only the patient but also her family. The management of the condition is usually entirely by the family doctor, though many specialists have an interest in various aspects of the syndrome.

Two groups of symptoms are frequently associated with menstruation—the premenstrual syndrome and dysmenorrhoea. Probably 20-40% of women have symptoms of the former disorder, of sufficient severity to be helped by treatment. Women who have had toxaemia of pregnancy have a high incidence of premenstrual symptoms. Age tends to increase the severity of the symptoms which often become a problem in the mid thirties.

Aetiology

Multiple factors are involved, some of which are still unknown. The time relationship of the symptoms to menstruation and the fact that they can continue after bilateral oophorectomy and hysterectomy suggests that cyclical changes in the hypothalamus, pituitary or adrenals may be the fundamental cause of the syndrome. There is some evidence that premenstrual sufferers have lower levels of progesterone during the luteal phase of the menstrual cycle.

Progesterone, in addition to its other functions, is an antagonist of aldosterone, as it can increase urinary sodium and chloride excretion in humans. It has been suggested that possible 'imbalance' of these corticoids occurring in a cyclical manner could account for the syndrome. Further evidence is needed before this can be considered other than a hypothesis.

Psychological factors may also be important. Premenstrual sufferers are more likely to have mothers who suffered painful menstruation, to be separated or divorced and dissatisfied with work. They also tend to to have higher anxiety and neuroticism scores and more negative attitudes to their bodies, genitals, sex and masturbation.

It is important to emphasize that premenstrual symptoms can be severe in 'normal' women and may be absent in neurotic women. In general, however, the incidence of the syndrome in neurotic women is 2-3 times that of a control group of women.

Symptoms

A very wide range of symptoms is covered by the term premenstrual syndrome. Most women experience symptoms in the week prior to menstruation which usually remit abruptly with the onset of menstruation. Occasionally patients also experience symptoms at the time of ovulation. It is the cyclical nature of the symptoms and their relationship to menstruation that is diagnostic of the disorder.

The commonest symptoms are tiredness, headaches, irritability, depression and swelling of the breasts and abdomen.

Tiredness

This can vary in severity but in general the woman finds it difficult to cope with routine jobs and feels tired and sleepy during the day.

Headaches

These are among the most common symptoms—they may range in severity from a mild headache relieved by aspirin to a true migraine with the usual aura, vertigo and vomiting. The headaches may last a few hours to several days.

Irritability

Irritability is an important symptom, particularly for the family. The patient is often unaware of the change in herself. She becomes intolerant, impatient and bad-tempered with her children and husband. Again, after menstruation the symptoms resolve rapidly.

Depression

This is an important, frequent symptom. Patients weep readily at this time and have a pessimistic outlook. These symptoms are more frequent in the menopausal woman. It has already been mentioned that suicidal attempts and suicide are more frequent at this time of the menstrual cycle.

Other Symptoms

Patients with some chronic medical condition, e.g. asthma, epilepsy, migraine, skin lesions, may all have an exacerbation of symptoms in the premenstrual phase of the cycle. Varicose veins may be more painful and prominent at this time.

Patients may have abdominal and breast swelling. Fluctuations of weight can occur at this time, but a definite correlation of water retention with the symptoms has not been uniformly found.

Diagnosis

Diagnosis of the premenstrual syndrome is not usually difficult, but memory is sometimes unreliable and it may be useful to ask the patient to record menstruation and symptoms for several cycles so that the relationship can be clearly seen.

Treatment

Not all patients with the symptoms require active treatment. Because of the diversity of symptoms there are a number of possible methods of treatment. In clinical practice one often finds that one line of treatment is effective for several months, but then symptoms become troublesome again and a different approach may be needed.

(1) General supportive treatment with an explanation of the symptoms to the patient (and her husband) is important, while water and salt restriction before the expected period may also be helpful.

(2) Placebo is known to be extremely effective in this condition, emphasizing the importance of psychological factors in therapy.

(3) Many women feel 'out of control' and benefit from learning new coping techniques, relaxation training and interventions which reduce environmental stress.

(4) *Endocrine treatment*

(a) Where symptoms are clearly related to the luteal phase it may be possible to suppress them by hormonal intervention. Some workers recommend progesterone, either by daily, intramuscular injections or an oral form such as dydrogesterone for the last 7-10 days of the menstrual cycle.

Suppression of the cycle with a progestogen given from day 5 to day 25 also tends to ameliorate symptoms.

(b) Bromergocryptine has been found effective, especially for cyclical breast symptoms.

(c) An aldosterone antagonist (spironolactone (Aldactone A) 25 mg. q.d.s.) for 10 days before the expected period is also effective in treating some patients with *severe* symptoms.

(d) Oral contraceptives given regularly can have a useful effect on premenstrual tension and dysmenorrhoea. However, some patients find side effects—weight increase and nausea—troublesome.

PSYCHIATRIC SYMPTOMS AND PREGNANCY

In the first few months of pregnancy depressive symptoms are not uncommon, particularly if the pregnancy is unwanted. As a rule these depressive symptoms are mild and correspond to those previously described as reactive depression. Occasionally, there are threats of suicide and the question of the psychiatric indications for termination of pregnancy may be raised. Usually if the patient is treated with supportive care, social help, and, if necessary, anti-depressive medication, symptoms settle by the 3rd or 4th month. Long lasting severe depression in pregnancy is a rarity, but, as has been mentioned in chapter 18, suicide in pregnancy does occur. Patients with schizophrenia or neurotic symptoms are in fact often remarkably well during their pregnancies.

The usual clinical problem about termination concerns the girl with personality problems (whose pregnancy may be a symptom of these). Termination is then one of the possible ways of management. Each individual patient needs detailed consideration, with due attention being paid to her personality resources, and the family setting. Termination may be judged to be the best way to help, but it is important to emphasize the value of continued psychiatric care throughout this time of crisis. The depressed middle-aged woman who becomes pregnant again after her family have grown up is another clinical situation when termination may be considered to be advisable on psychiatric grounds. Again the whole family situation needs to be considered. In regard to termination of pregnancy students must, by discussion, come to understand their own position on the range of opinions that at one end give the mother the decision, and at the other that termination is only allowable for very concrete medical reasons.

Post partum psychiatric symptoms are also frequent and sometimes these can be severe. Mild depressive symptoms are relatively frequent and have been reported to occur after 30% of pregnancies ('post-partum blues'). However, they are not usually long lasting and respond well to supportive care. There is no definite correlation between these symptoms and age, length of marriage, parity, course of delivery and lactation.

Severe psychiatric symptoms are less common; they usually develop within 1-3 weeks of delivery and often begin suddenly with the patient developing ideas that people are talking about her or are trying to poison her. Sometimes the picture is clearly a schizophrenic one from the start; in others severe depressive symptoms occur which either persist or are followed, in some patients, by definite thought disorder and auditory hallucinations. The cause of these severe post partum psychiatric disturbances is unknown, but their time of onset suggests some unknown metabolic factors. These patients usually need to be admitted to a psychiatric hospital where, whether the symptoms are schizophrenic or depressive, good results are usually obtained from a prolonged course of E.C.T. These patients stand about a 1 in 10 chance of developing similar symptoms at the next pregnancy.

THE MENOPAUSE

The menopause is the time that menstruation ceases. The climacteric refers to the period before and after the actual cessation of menstruation, during which time there is a waning of endocrine activity. In considering the causes of menopausal symptoms one must look further than oestrogen withdrawal.

In women at this time there are often marked social and psychological changes taking place. The children are leaving or have left home, her husband is usually engrossed in his own work problems, and she finds that no one is dependent on her. In addition the problems of growing old, losing her appearance and the routine of household duties all are all important.

Men also have a mid-life crisis; but overt problems present at a somewhat later age, when they have to retire from active employment.

Incidence of Menopausal Symptoms

There are very marked differences in reports ranging from claims that '70% of women have symptoms' to claims that '70% of women do not have symptoms'.

Psychiatric Symptoms

Depressive symptoms (see chapter 12), *anxiety and other neurotic symptoms* (see chapter 10) are the important ones and will not be described again here. Paranoid symptoms are not uncommon.

Vasomotor Symptoms

Vasomotor symptoms—characteristically 'hot flushes' are common and vary considerably in frequency and severity.

Other Complaints

In addition, headaches, arthralgia, hypertension, diabetes and obesity are all frequent problems at this time.

Treatment

Many women have some of the symptoms mentioned above but do not seek medical advice, accepting them as something that will settle in time.

It is probably true that women who have suffered in the past from neurotic or depressive symptoms are likely to have further symptoms at the menopause. Sexual difficulties need to be asked about as they are not uncommon at this time. Supportive care for all medical, psychiatric and social problems is important. In this regard some women find that taking employment outside the home is particularly helpful once their children are independent.

As a rule oestrogens (e.g. ethinyloestradiol 0·01-0·05 mg. per day) are helpful in relieving vasomotor symptoms and may also help associated psychological symptoms. Supportive care, social change and anti-anxiety or anti-depressant drugs may be needed.

SUMMARY

The premenstrual syndrome is a frequent cause of symptoms. Tiredness, headaches, irritability and depression are the main symptoms. Principles of treatment are described.

Attention is drawn to mild depressive symptoms often seen in early pregnancy and following delivery. Problems of termination are discussed.

The severe psychiatric syndrome that occasionally follows pregnancy is usually characterized by schizophrenic symptoms and responds well to a prolonged course of electroconvulsive therapy.

Psychiatric symptoms associated with the menopause are described. An integrated approach to management is needed to consider the relative roles of biological, psychological and social factors for each woman.

REFERENCES

Dalton, K., *The Premenstrual Syndrome.* William Heinemann (London, 1964). A comprehensive account of all aspects of this disorder.

Dennerstein, L., 'The Menopause', in *Gynaecology, Sex and Psyche*, ed. Dennerstein, L., Burrows, G. D., Cox, L. and Wood, C. (Melbourne University Press, 1978).

Pitt, B., *Mid Life Crisis.* Sheldon Press (London, 1980). A useful overview of middle life problems of men and women.

23

SEXUAL PROBLEMS

Patients who complain of sexual problems (e.g. masturbation, impotence, frigidity, homosexuality) often present a problem to the family doctor, mainly because he has had little or no training as a student which will help him to understand and treat these complaints.

The first clinical fact to emphasize is that these 'sexual problems' are extremely common. Sometimes it is the wife or husband who wants treatment for their spouse. Sometimes sexual complaints are the first indication of schizophrenia or depression. Impotence may be the first sign of organic disease (but rarely is). Sometimes the presentation of such problems may indicate that the person is in danger of legal or police action. Usually the sexual problem has been present for many years, and one must find out *why this patient has come for help at this particular time.*

An important difficulty with sexual problems is the question of 'what is normal'? There are two common ways of using this word:

An 'ideal' concept of normal, where we may believe that the 'normal' adult male should be completely heterosexual, be married to one wife and have two children.

There is also a statistical concept of normality. Here no *value judgements* are made about what is normal sexual behaviour. Instead, enquiries are made to see what are the facts about sexual behaviour in a given community. In this respect Kinsey's studies have given some information about the sexual behaviour of groups of men and women in America. Here normality is a matter of measurement. One needs to go even further than this and consider patterns of sexual behaviour as seen in different parts of the world today (and in the past) and to relate it to sexual behaviour in other species. Such a review is provided by Ford and Beach (1951). It is quite clear from their findings that what our society considers abnormal sexual behaviour is considered normal in other societies now and in the past. It may be argued that this is not relevant to medical practice in Western society, yet some notion of 'social relativity' is necessary.

Even in one society, as Kinsey has shown, the sexual behaviour of people in Social Classes 1 and 5 may be quite different. Doctors in Social Class 1 should therefore be aware of these 'normal' differences in most of their patients. Students are advised to read the above reference so that these notions can be understood.

EVALUATION OF SEXUAL PROBLEMS

A careful assessment is necessary. This involves assessment of the patient and the partner, individually and together. During this evaluation the doctor aims at identifying the following:

(1) What are the presenting complaints and their duration? Have these problems always been present or are they of more recent onset?

(2) What is the aetiology of these complaints? Are the complaints symptomatic of an underlying problem such as depression or an organic illness or marital disharmony or do they appear to be a learned pattern of response? Are there conflicts about sexuality present?

(3) What approach to therapy is likely to be the most helpful?

In general where a cause is present therapy should be directed to the cause. Behavioural techniques are very effective for those problems which seem to be learned patterns of behaviour. Psychotherapy is sometimes needed to resolve conflicts about sexuality.

The other therapy decision is whether to treat an individual or the couple. Individual therapy is recommended when the patient has not fully accepted his or her own sexuality and is uncomfortable about looking at or exploring the genitalia. Once conflicts about sexuality have been resolved and the genitalia accepted, a conjoint approach to therapy is to be preferred.

This approach was developed by Masters and Johnson, who highlighted the fact that sexual inadequacy exists within a relationship and there is no such thing as an uninvolved partner. This method of therapy focuses on the sexual interaction of the couple. Masters and Johnson developed a programme of pleasuring and communication exercises called 'sensate focus'. These exercises help desensitize the couple to the sexual situation.

Free discussions between the partners is encouraged and marital difficulties both sexual and non-sexual are ventilated. The couple are then instructed to spend 30 minutes a day for the next week in non-genital pleasuring. The partners should be naked and the room illuminated.

After the next interview when further discussions are promoted, genital pleasuring should take place each night for the next week but ejaculation and orgasms should not be produced. Constant verbal and non-verbal feedback by the couple must take place. After the third interview, coitus should occur after prolonged pleasuring. For women with orgasmic failure training in clitoral stimulation is an important part of the method of training.

For further details of this approach students should read the references at the end of this chapter.

HOMOSEXUALITY

The problems of homosexuality will be discussed to illustrate the general psychiatric approach to sexual problems. Homosexuality is common in men and women in our society. One man in 20 is a practising homosexual. In women the frequency is probably about half this figure. Most homosexuals do not seek medical advice and most are effective members of our society. Contrary to general opinion, male homosexuals are not as a rule interested sexually in pre-pubertal boys and tend to despise those who are.

Culture

Ford and Beach reported that 49 out of 76 primitive societies accept homosexual activity; other tribes do not and punish such behaviour. Some animals appear bisexual.

Incidence

Homosexuality is not an all-or-none phenomenon. Kinsey in his studies used a scale which graded his subjects' homosexual behaviour:

0— exclusively heterosexual

1—⎫
2—⎭ predominantly heterosexual (e.g. as temporary behaviour in prisoners and P.O.W.)

3— equally hetero and homosexual

4—⎫
5—⎭ predominantly homosexual

6— exclusively homosexual

Four per cent of Kinsey's male sample were in category 6, while one-third had had some homosexual interests.

Female homosexuality (lesbianism) is also widespread, and a similar scale is applicable.

Homosexuality is seen in all social classes and professions; and in people with all types of physique and personality. Generalizations about the physical and psychological make up of homosexual men and women have no validity. The effeminate group of male homosexuals is a minority 'non-typical' group.

Aetiology

The real problem is the exclusively homosexual person who cannot have an erotic relationship with someone of the opposite sex. There is no chromosomal abnormality; no genetic hypothesis is tenable. No endocrine abnormalities are found.

More is known about male homosexuality than lesbianism. Some studies have shown that affected males are late in the birth order and are commonly born to older mothers.

It is inappropriate to use an 'illness model' in considering homosexuality.

Psychopathology

Freud suggested that there was too intense and exclusive a relationship with the mother. There develops severe guilt feelings with fantasies of punishment by castration. These wishes and fears are repressed, but with further sexual development the male homosexual avoids sex with women because of these repressed complexes.

Studies of groups of homosexual men and their parents have shown that there is usually an intense relationship with the mother and an unsatisfactory one with the father, who may be a weak, indifferent figure. Paternal deprivation is more frequent than in control patients. The mother is often a demanding, overprotective, domineering woman. There may be a rigid suppression of mention of all things sexual in the family, and mothers may even occasionally encourage the boy to play and dress like a girl.

Diagnosis

A diagnosis of exclusive homosexuality should not be made before the age of 25. In adolescence, transitory homosexual feelings and behaviour are not infrequent and they can cause great distress to the individual.

Treatment

In general, treatment is directed towards the problems raised by homosexuality and not towards the disorder itself.

In this regard long term supportive care is helpful. In adolescence, acceptance and support are of particular importance. As has been mentioned, at this age sexual orientation can change. Again it should be emphasized that homosexuals may not seek medical advice unless some particular problems have developed. In our society, for men this is often the threat of police action. Paranoid symptoms are frequent in homosexuals in our society and may need treatment. Other patients may in fact be presenting because of depressive symptoms.

PSYCHIATRIC REFERRAL

It may well be that the problem will be found to be too complex and the patient should be referred for psychiatric advice. In this respect patients who seek help for transvestism (cross dressing); fetishism (sexual stimulation from an inanimate object—usually an article of clothing); exhibitionism, or any masochistic or sadistic sexual practices are best referred. So too should transexualists—patients who want to change their sex. Homosexuals who seek help are also best referred to a psychiatrist. Husbands and wives who seek help together about sexual problems may either respond to advice and management or may be extremely difficult to manage. If it appears that one or both partners has a pronounced personality abnormality or marked neurotic symptoms, the family doctor might be well advised to refer these patients for further management. Mention has already been made about the difficulties that can arise if the untrained doctor attempts 'psychotherapy' in patients with sexual problems (chapter 11).

SUMMARY

The doctor's usual difficulties in dealing with sexual problems are discussed.

Sexual problems should be considered from a wide biological, social and historical view point.

The aetiology and management of homosexuality is discussed.

Some common problems of sexual dysfunction within a relationship are discussed. 'Why has this patient come for help now?' is a key question to answer clinically with sexual problems.

Suggestions are made about the sorts of sexual problems to refer to psychiatrists.

REFERENCES

Clarke, M., 'Treating frigidity means treating the couple', *Australian Medical Journal*, vol. 2 (1974), pp. 405-9.

Dennerstein, L., Burrows, G. D., Cox, L. and Wood, C., *Gynaecology, Sex and Psyche* (Melbourne University Press, 1978). An introduction to the subject, specially written for medical students.

Ford, C. S. and Beach, F. A., *Patterns of Sexual Behaviour*. Harper & Row (New York, 1970). Summarizes a large amount of data from anthropological and biological studies of sexual behaviour.

Masters, W. H. and Johnson, V. E., *Human Sexual Response*. Little, Brown (Boston, 1966).

Masters, W. H. and Johnson, V. E., *Human Sexual Inadequacy*. Little, Brown (Boston, 1970).

Storr, A., *Sexual Deviation*. Pelican, 1974. A useful account of these problems.

West, D. J., *Homosexuality*. Pelican (Harmondsworth, 1974). The best short account of homosexuality.

24

SOME ASPECTS OF SOCIAL PSYCHIATRY

In recent years the application of the methods of study used by social scientists to medical problems has been of great interest. The study of the complex relationship between the sociologists' findings on the one hand and the doctor's on the other is the field of *Social Medicine*. In particular, sociologists have contributed significantly to the understanding of the aetiology, prevention and treatment of certain illnesses. They have also studied the effect of illnesses on the family and in industry. This approach is still unfamiliar to most medical students, yet it can claim to add an important new dimension to medical thinking. Such studies have been of particular relevance to psychiatry, comprising the field of *social psychiatry* which investigates both the *social causes* of psychiatric illness and the *social effects* of such illness.

PREVALENCE OF PSYCHIATRIC ILLNESSES

Some of the basic aspects of social psychiatry—the incidence and prevalence of psychiatric illness—have already been reviewed in chapter 3. It is clear that neurosis, personality disorders and psychosomatic illnesses are frequent, important problems in present day Western society; but it is difficult to ascertain to what extent these problems occur in other societies—e.g. in Africa or Asia. Reliable comparisons cannot be made about the incidence of psychiatric illnesses in different parts of the world today, particularly with these less severe forms of illness. Comparisons between hospital admissions in different countries of the severe disorders may also be invalid because of the different social criteria for hospital admission and the availability of psychiatric services.

Studies of psychiatric disorders in different cultures show clearly that culture shapes the clinical pattern of many illnesses, though the fundamental features of an illness like schizophrenia can be recognized throughout the world.

Perhaps the most interesting studies in different cultures are the effects of different child rearing habits on subsequent personality development. Studies in this important field are however only beginning.

The question of whether there has been an increase in psychiatric illness over the years is difficult to answer. Goldhammer and Marshall studied the admission rates to Massachusetts Mental Hospitals from 1840 to 1940. They found that despite the very marked changes that had occurred in New England society there was no appreciable difference in the admission rates for people under fifty years of age. Increases in admission rates were found in patients over 50 but people now live longer and elderly people with psychiatric illness are more readily referred to psychiatric hospitals. Thus as regards severe psychiatric illness, there is no evidence from this study of any increase in rate, despite the changes in modern society. However, there is no way of making a similar comparison with neurosis, as no figures of incidence in the past are available and even today incidence figures of neurosis vary widely.

SOCIAL CAUSES OF ILLNESS

It is common to read in popular books on psychology and psychiatry that civilized Western society is to blame for the large number of people with neuroses and also for the individuals in our society who repeatedly break the law. More particularly, economic pressures, marriage and divorce laws and the upbringing of children are incriminated as causative factors in the aetiology of psychiatric illness. Is it possible to study these notions? There is in North America a Protestant sect—the Hutterites—who live in colonies in certain farming areas. The sect believes in common ownership; there are no wages, birth control or divorce. Families usually have several children. The sect uses modern farming methods, while schooling and medicine are on the American pattern. Anecdotal evidence suggested that the Hutterites were free from psychiatric illness and this was claimed to be due to the absence of financial stress, family dissention and competition between peers.

Eaton and Weil made a detailed survey of the Hutterites and found that, in fact, psychiatric illnesses of all severity did occur among the Hutterites. There were differences however between the Hutterites and the American population, in the absence of murder, assaults and juvenile delinquency. Alcoholism and drug addiction were rare. These findings point to the importance of social causes in considering the aetiology of these last conditions. The authors conclude 'our findings do not confirm the hypothesis that a simple and relatively uncomplicated way of life provides immunity from mental disorders'.

This is the sort of study that tries to correlate sociological findings on the one hand and psychiatric findings on the other.

SOCIAL CLASS AND PSYCHIATRIC ILLNESS

People who work can be grouped in our society into a number of social classes that depend essentially on their economic status and educational background. These groups are not static but, in medicine, studies of differences in the incidence of certain illnesses in certain social classes and occupations have helped our understanding of the aetiology of these illnesses (e.g. cardiac infarction, peptic ulceration). Similar studies have been of interest in psychiatry. It has been shown that schizophrenia is 5 times as frequent in Social Classes 4 and 5 (manual workers, unskilled labourers) than in 1 and 2 (professional and white collar workers). Schizophrenics, too, tend to live in densely populated city areas of low economic status. These findings could mean either:

(1) that conditions in certain areas of cities and certain occupations tend to favour the development of schizophrenia, or

(2) patients with schizophrenia tend to drift to these areas of the city and because of their illness are untrained and take jobs in Social Classes 4 and 5.

Investigations have been carried out in Britain and in America to study these alternative interpretations. The evidence shows that the second 'drift' hypothesis is the more likely.

It has been mentioned that social class groupings are not static. The individual person may move upwards or downwards in the social class groupings. Such *socially mobile* people are likely to encounter many problems in such movement. The 'upward mobile' is likely to be an ambitious person striving for success. It is among this group of people that certain psychosomatic illnesses are found to be particularly frequent.

Hollingshead and Redlich in their study in New Haven showed that the sort of treatment received by patients with psychiatric illnesses is related to the social class of the patient. More general social factors can also affect psychiatric treatment: in some countries today certain forms of treatment are not allowed (e.g. leucotomy) while, in others, Freud's books are not available.

MARRIAGE AND PSYCHIATRIC ILLNESS

It has been shown that the social factor of marriage and the diagnosis of schizophrenia have a low statistical correlation. What explanations are possible for this finding?

(1) a single person with schizophrenia is more readily admitted to a hospital than a married schizophrenic,

(2) in married life there are certain factors which protect against schizophrenia,

(3) people who develop schizophrenia have previous personality difficulties which make marriage unlikely,

(4) the illness, coming on as it usually does in adolescence, interferes with the normal social behaviour at this age which culminates in marriage.

Investigations have shown that the latter two explanations are the most relevant. When observations like the above have been shown unequivocally, the next stage is a number of discrete investigations to study the alternative explanations for the observations.

MIGRATION AND PSYCHIATRIC ILLNESS

Other interesting studies concerning sociology and psychiatry relate to migration. Migrants have a high rate of psychiatric illness. Is this: (1) because of the stresses involved in living in a new country, or (2) were they ill or abnormal before they migrated?

Studies of migrants to the United States from Scandinavian countries show that the second hypothesis explained the observations best.

Studies of the incidence of psychiatric illnesses in migrant groups to Australia have provided some interesting information. In one study, first admissions to State psychiatric hospitals and outpatient clinics were analysed. It was found that the incidence of schizophrenia was higher in non-British migrants, especially in Eastern Europeans, compared with Australian and British-born people. The incidence of alcoholism was highest among the Australian born and Britons. Personality disorders among adolescent migrants were more frequent than in the Australian population, except for adolescents from Southern Europe.

SUICIDE

As regards suicide, certain countries have quite different suicide rates, e.g. Japan with a high one and Spain with a low one. Certain occupations (doctors, students) have high suicide rates while others (farmers and clergymen) have low rates. It is also a well known fact that suicide and social isolation are related (see chapter 18).

SOCIAL EFFECTS OF PSYCHIATRIC DISORDERS

The 'other half' of social psychiatry concerns the effects of psychiatric illness on society. Most research in this field has concentrated on the family of patients—some investigations looking at possible pathological family influences, and others the effects of severe psychiatric illness on children of the patients. The difficulties of sorting out cause and effect are very great in these studies, as is the difficulty of sorting out hereditary and environmental factors.

Other investigations have studied the effect of psychiatric illness in industry. The effect of a psychiatric disorder in one individual can have a profound effect throughout the world, e.g. an assassination by a paranoid person. The number of crimes that are associated with psychiatric illness is another important field of study. The social effects of alcoholism have been described in chapter 17.

MATERNAL DEPRIVATION

These studies originated in the work of Bowlby who found that children who were deprived of their mother (by death, separation, severe illness) particularly between 6 months and 2 years of age, developed enduring abnormalities in personality structure not only in the emotional, but also in the intellectual field. The incidence of juvenile delinquency in children so deprived is high.

Many investigations have been and are being done in this field of study involving not only human, but also animal studies. It is certain that not all children so deprived develop abnormally; much obviously depends on the 'mother substitute' and the events which led to the deprivation. It is also true that any abnormalities which develop are not necessarily permanent and the crucial time for deprivation to be pathogenic is still in dispute.

Despite this, Bowlby's work has led to a great deal of research on the whole problem of parent-child interaction.

In clinical psychiatric practice the adult who, as a child, has been brought up in a number of foster homes or orphanages, who has been in remand homes and later in prison, who cannot make a satisfactory marriage, or be a competent parent is commonly encountered.

The effects of paternal deprivation on the sexual behaviour of boys is also a recent research interest, a high incidence of homosexuality being found when these boys reach adult life.

SUMMARY

The field of social psychiatry is defined and certain investigations mentioned that illustrate how some of the problems in this field are tackled.

REFERENCES

Ainsworth, M. et al., *Deprivation of Maternal Care: A reassessment of its effects.* W. H. O. Public Health Papers no. 14 (Geneva, 1962).

Bowlby, J., *Maternal Care and Mental Health.* W. H. O. Monograph Series no. 2 (Geneva, 1951). An account of the effects of maternal deprivation.

Garrad, J. and Rosenheim, M., *Social Aspects of Clinical Medicine.* Baillière, Tindall & Cassell (London, 1970). The best practical small book on this subject for students.

Packard, V., *The Status Seekers.* Longmans (London, 1960). Students unfamiliar with sociological methods and findings might find this 'readable' book of value. The chapters that deal with differences in behaviour of different social classes are important for doctors.

Susser, M. W. and Watson, W. *Sociology in Medicine.* Oxford University Press, 2nd edn 1977. This book is a good introduction to the problems of sociology in medicine.

25

SOME ASPECTS OF LEGAL PSYCHIATRY

Students need to know little about the details of the complex issues which can arise when psychiatry and the law have a common problem. A doctor's usual contact with these issues is the occasional certification procedure. *In general, most patients with psychiatric illness can be treated informally,* i.e. they can be admitted to hospital in the same way as patients with physical illness, the patient being willing to accept the medical help offered.

All countries have laws whereby a patient with a psychiatric illness who needs medical attention, and who may be a danger to himself or others but is unwilling to enter hospital can be forced to do so. Certification is usually by one or two qualified doctors (in some countries a magistrate is also involved). Once admitted to a psychiatric hospital, the psychiatrists there can extend the certification order until the patient has responded to treatment.

In Victoria, at present, the general practitioner or any medically qualified practitioner (not an employee of the Mental Health Authority) has to describe the main symptoms suggesting a psychiatric illness on a special form. In addition, he should obtain a signed request from the nearest relative who is seeking hospital treatment for the patient. (If no relative is available, a policeman often completes this request). The patient is then taken to the hospital, either by taxi with the relative, or by the police. Once admitted, the psychiatrist superintendent examines the patient and endorses the request order if clinically appropriate. The order may be renewed within 21 days by the psychiatrists at the hospital.

Suicidal attempts are not, in most places, now considered a matter for legal intervention.

The problems of 'insanity' as a defence in the courts of law will not be discussed in detail here. If a doctor is asked to give an opinion about the psychiatric state of a person who is to be tried for some legal offence, he would be wise to try and leave the matter to a qualified psychiatrist. If this cannot be done, it is essential that a most complete psychiatric history should be taken, not only from the subject, but also from relatives and police. Several interviews with the subject are also needed before any firm conclusions are made.

The family doctor is however unlikely to be involved with these psychiatric issues. He will encounter the problems presented by juvenile delinquency, but details about this important subject can be found in the book recommended below. Again the total psychological, physical and social approach to the problem, emphasized throughout these notes, is the most helpful.

SUMMARY

Most patients with psychiatric illness can be treated informally. Certification procedures are necessary for the few patients who refuse treatment and may be a danger to themselves or others.

REFERENCES

Bovet, L., *Psychiatric Aspects of Juvenile Delinquency*. W.H.O. Monograph Series no. 1 (Geneva, 1951). A lucid statement of our knowledge of an important social problem.

Wiley, H. J. and Stallworthy, K. R., *Mental Abnormality and the Law*. N. M. Peryer (Christchurch, N.Z., 1962). A balanced account of the subject.

26

CONSULTATION–LIAISON PSYCHIATRY

Students will spend some time clerking on patients in the general hospital referred to the psychiatric services. This chapter (and chapters 13 and 14) aim to help students with this task.

The field of consultation–liaison psychiatry is one of increasing importance. The consultation is where the psychiatrist is asked to assess and advise treatment for a particular patient under the care of another specialist. The term 'liaison psychiatry' implies a rather broader function. In some hospitals, and in some units, particularly those that deal with intensive care, nephrology, oncology and rehabilitation, psychiatrists have become members of the particular 'team'. It is in these areas that the complexities of medical care can lead us to forget firstly that the 'patient' is a person and secondly that doctors and nurses have their own personalities and personal problems. Often the psychiatrists' role is to ventilate staff conflicts and problems, but they also bring to the liaison field a knowledge of the individuals' and families' coping mechanisms. Students should become aware of the individual patients and the particular family's response to physical illnesses.

Psychiatric morbidity is often unrecognized in general hospital patients. Surveys have shown that about 50 per cent of 'new' medical and 20 per cent of 'new' surgical patients have significant psychiatric symptoms. In the wards some 30–60 per cent of patients will be found to have similar problems. In one study in a medical ward, 43 out of 150 patients were found to have significant depressive symptoms. Only 2 had been referred for psychiatric treatment and only 6 case notes mentioned any of the depressive symptoms.

Student Clerking

The principles of history taking and mental state examination have already been described. In consultation work, students should adopt a more *'problem orientated approach'* than when in the psychiatric wards.

Students should define the *presenting problem* as clearly as possible with information from doctors, nurses and relatives. *Acute brain syndromes* (chapter 15) and *depressive symptoms* (chapter 12) are particularly common and the *presence* or *absence* of key symptoms of the syndromes need to be formally defined. *Alcohol consumption* must be inquired into and an informant asked about this. The 25 questions listed in Appendix 6 can be used as a self-administered screening test; scores of more than 7 indicate that the individual could be an alcoholic, and further assessment is indicated. The use of other drugs also needs careful inquiry.

In the.*mental state* examination special attention must be paid to orientation, memory, depression and anxiety. In regard to orientation it has been emphasized in chapter 15 that the symptoms of an acute organic brain syndrome can fluctuate markedly throughout the twenty-four hours. Careful recording of answers to questions on orientation may need to be made several times a day.

The problems of making a positive diagnosis of psychological symptoms are discussed on page 51.

As well as the problem orientated approach, students must aim to understand *what sort of person is this patient?* What was *the life situation* before admission to hospital? In this regard it often helps to ask how the patients spent a typical day before the hospital admission.

Students must listen to the patient and aim to see at least one of the relatives or friends. The effect of the illness on the 'nearest and dearest' should be assessed. Who visits? How often? What happens?

It is also useful to attempt to define the *patient's personality* features, because it may be relevant to behaviour in hospital. Five common personality patterns are the orderly, controlled obsessive; the dependent over-demanding; the dramatizing emotionally involved; the long suffering, self sacrificing; and the guarded, querulous, suspicious patient.

In the *physical examination* special attention should be paid to the presence or absence of a fever and the presence or absence of respiratory and urinary tract infection. Cardiac failure must be looked for and the C.N.S. examined closely. Alcoholism, thyroid disease, Parkinson's disease, and subdural haematomas must be considered almost routinely with each patient.

COPING BEHAVIOUR AND CRISIS THEORY

How are individuals able to cope with the pain and suffering of severe physical illness?

Students will be familiar with the notions of *physiological homeostasis* and how the body attempts to maintain this. Individuals also need a *psychological and social homeostasis.* When some particular stress is met, the individual employs his own habitual ways of coping. If the stress is severe, then the habitual responses may be inadequate and feelings of severe anxiety and guilt occur. Over days, weeks or months some equilibrium is re-established.

CRISIS THEORY looks at the ways that major crises are coped with. A person with *acute severe physical illness* faces separation from family and friends, loss of a key role in life, permanent changes in bodily functions, assault on self image and self esteem, distress, anxiety, guilt, anger, hopelessness and the uncertain future. Patients are more receptive to outside influences at this time e.g. it is at such times that a cognitive attempt to give up nicotine or alcohol can be made at the doctor's suggestion.

Patients admitted to hospital with physical illnesses have to deal not only with discomfort and incapacity but also with the hospital environment and special treatment procedures. Separation from family and friends is a problem for all patients but a particularly important one for children.

A patient with *chronic physical illness* has to learn to accept *increased dependency* and *limitation in functional abilities*. Acceptance of disability is the first and most important psychological task. The family problems that arise when a child develops a chronic physical illness have been a particular focus for study.

A patient with a *fatal illness* has to cope with management of his own anxiety and despair, the maintenance of self esteem and the mourning of the people and objects he is losing. One source of anxiety is that the bodily changes and loss of functions will make his family and friends reject him. The family reaction of shock, denial, grief, anger, resentment all need to be understood. This very important area is discussed elsewhere (pages 87-8).

These and other problems are reviewed in the book and articles mentioned below. The book containing personal experiences of illness, written often by doctor patients, is an important one.

SUMMARY

In consultation–liaison clerking students should adopt a problem orientated approach. Depression, acute brain syndromes and alcoholism must be considered in every patient. The psychological responses of the patient and the family to acute, chronic and fatal physical illnesses need to be understood.

REFERENCES

Moos, R. H. (ed.), *Coping with Physical Illness.* Plenum Publishers (New York, 1977). A useful review of coping theories and their application to medical practice.

Lipowski, Z. J., *Review of Consultation Psychiatry and Psychosomatic Medicine* (1967).

Psychosomatic Medicine (1967) 29; 153-71
29; 201-24
29; 395-422

A detailed review of Consultation-Liaison Psychiatry.

Disabilities and how to live with them. The Lancet Limited (London, 1952). An important book describing personal experiences with severe illnesses.

CHILD PSYCHIATRY

by WINSTON RICKARDS

M.D , B.SC., F.R.A.C.P., F.A.N.Z.C.P., F.R.C.PSYCH., A.B.PS.S., M.A.PS.S., D.P.M.

Director, Department of Psychiatry, Royal Children's Hospital

Senior Associate in Child Psychiatry, Department of Psychiatry, University of Melbourne

27

PRINCIPLES OF CHILD DEVELOPMENT

The child psychiatrist is concerned with individual children and particular families in their changing society. He must understand the child and parents, and how they function as a family in their culture and must have special knowledge of child development.

Each child is born with a potential *individual* to him. The extent to which this potential will be realized depends not only upon his genetic endowment but also on environmental experiences. There is a wide range of individual differences in children: e.g. temperamental differences can be observed in infants that persist through early childhood.

Development is characterized by various stages, each showing predominant levels of organization from which the next stage unfolds.

From conception, there is a constant interaction between the infant and the environment. While the intra-uterine milieu permits growth until the infant can survive, damage *in utero* from a variety of factors, such as rubella, can affect the foetus.

The birth process itself presents hazards. Birth trauma can produce gross or subtle defects; it may also serve as a source of anxiety, fear and guilt for the mother and affect her emotional freedom to nurse the baby.

The child matures through the phases of (1) infant, (2) toddler, (3) pre-school child, (4) school-age child, (5) adolescent. In healthy children there are wide norms, spurts, and lags in the growth process. Development is subject to maturational variations and can be affected by environmental factors such as inappropriate stimulation or deprivation.

Relationships

The child's first relationship is to the mother or mother figure who supplies his needs, and is the first object of his awareness. Subsequent development involves an increasingly complex series of relationships with other people.

As a *toddler* he relates to siblings and others within the family while as a *pre-school child*, relationships outside the family with *peers and other adults* continue the socialization process.

The *school-age child* is presented with a task-oriented situation—a social structure which is the prototype of future society where he must relate to teachers, cope socially, and strive competitively with fellow pupils and settle to the task of learning.

The *adolescent* is presented with the complexities of sexuality and adult identification and role within his peer group.

Socialization from infancy involves the establishment of *meaningful and adequate relationships* through a series of stages, each of which is influenced by the way in which the previous stage has been accomplished.

This principle is fundamental to the understanding of development. Physical, intellectual and emotional growth proceed through well-defined developmental phases, each stage depending upon the successful resolution of the previous stage.

At each phase the child shows *characteristic responses to stress*. For example: the *infant's* responses to stress are manifested physically with crying, vomiting, rocking, sleep disturbances, refusal of food, disorders of motility and retardation.

The *toddler* with his newly developed capacity for independence (e.g. walking) finds control difficult, and may show aggression to self, to people, and to objects by temper tantrums and hyperactivity. Under stress he may lose some of his newly-acquired skills and regress to earlier patterns of behaviour.

The *pre-school child* (2½ to 5 years) is characterized by the development of cognitive functions such as perception and speech. He has a rich fantasy life and egocentric, animistic thinking emerges with prelogical notions of causality. More obvious sexual identification develops, and social relationships with peers and adults widen. Under stress he may regress, or fail to develop socially, physically, intellectually and emotionally. His play may become constricted, stereotyped, or disorganized. Fears and guilt appear and phobic and obsessional symptoms may become evident.

The *early school-age child* (5 to 8 years) can tolerate separation from his parents and family without undue anxiety; he develops increasing independence and creativity, and is more secure in his sexual identification. His level of development should be such that he can channel aggressive and sexual drives into emotionally satisfying and socially acceptable outlets. This presumes that he has acquired bodily control over speech, sphincters and activity and that he can settle and attend to the teacher and the task. Under stress, anxiety may be shown by hyperactivity, short attention span, distractibility, impulsiveness, emotional lability and aggression. On the other hand his psychological defences are becoming more complex at this time, and the more traditional clinical psychiatric conditions can emerge, becoming more clearly defined as development proceeds.

The *adolescent* experiences intensification of sexual and aggressive impulses, increasing anxiety and problems relating to dependence and independence. Relationships with adults are characterized by rapidly fluctuating emotions of love and hate, dependence and attempted independence, while he constantly questions his values and ideals. Relationships with his peers and the choice of a vocation are added stresses in his attempts to achieve personal identity.

167

MOTHERING

The experience of mothering represents a biological, psychological and social crisis for the individual. Physical and emotional health, and appropriate psychological understanding and social circumstances are all necessary conditions for successful parenthood. The important issue is the mother's capacity to relate to her children, and to the particular child's specific needs at specific times.

Her maturity and preparedness for pregnancy, her health and psychological readiness at the time are important for the acceptance of the child; following the birth, in Winnicott's terms 'the ordinary devoted mother' can learn to read the child's cues, recognize his signals and respond intuitively.

Every child is a 'new experiment in nature' for the mother, and the particular relationship she establishes may be different in quality (often dramatically so), from her relationships with her other children. While her standard of care may appear to remain constant, skilled observation may reveal wide extremes in her emotional relationship with the child. Anxiety, guilt, fear and anger may stem from factors within herself or be activated by her current life experiences, such as stress within the family, and by the child's own behaviour.

The mother perceives and responds to the child with particular feelings which are influenced by past and present needs, activated during the ante-natal period, the birth experience and by current events. In the 'mature response', the mother can permit healthy growth of the child and respond realistically to his needs and behaviour. However, the emotionally disturbed parent may relate unrealistically to the child's needs and behaviour, because of her own unconsciously determined fears and guilts. The child may then be influenced or even moulded by maternal attitudes and behaviour which conflict sharply with his own innately determined behavioural patterns.

Just as the child responds to stress with symptoms, so the mother may respond not only with anxiety symptoms but also with distorted maternal responses. This is particularly so when *behaviour at certain stages of the child's development* arouses anxiety, leading to mutual emotional distress in mother and child. For example, the toddler's problems of hyperactivity, sphincter control, aggressive behaviour and independence may be too much for an obsessional mother who has managed to cope until that time.

It is important to realize that a mother can behave in an emotionally illogical way with her children and yet maintain an appearance of adjustment in her general behaviour.

Besides studying the child and mother as individuals, current research and clinical practice *studies the interaction* (*the transactional relationship*) and evaluates the contribution of child *and* mother.

THE FAMILY

While emphasis has been placed on the mother-child bond because of its importance in the establishment of the child's early object relations and its life-long significance, the importance of father should not be underestimated, and the same principles apply.

The Family as a Unit

It is useful to regard the family, like the individual, as a unit which has biological, psychological and social attributes. The family is conceived, grows and develops, adapts, has developmental crises and must find techniques of coping with stress and achieving an identity.

Factors Within the Family

Individuals in their lives assume many roles. In these different roles they need different skills. For instance, a successful businessman may be respected by his community, be a competent husband, but still fail to relate and provide healthy models for identification for his children. Individuals, while being relatively healthy within themselves, may break down in their *relationships* with others. Pressures of marriage and family life may highlight the dependence of members of the family with an unhealthy involvement of parents or grandparents.

Sickness provides a natural experiment which tests a family's resources. The presence of a disturbed or handicapped member, such as a retarded or physically handicapped child, is felt throughout the family and may be a stimulus for more cohesive behaviour or may precipitate disruption.

The *presenting patient* may not be the most disturbed member of the family. He is often an *'emissary in disguise'* for the emotionally disturbed family who seek help through a particular member. In the case of a child, sometimes the referral may be to control, punish or mould his behaviour to the family, or he may be the scapegoat behind which the family hides.

'Family process' is now an extensive area of current research. 'Driving the other person crazy' is a humorous way of referring to the types of communication and relationships seen in families of schizophrenic patients, and may be crucial to the understanding and effective management of the individual. The concept of a 'psychopathogenic carrier' in families arose when studies revealed that a clinically undiagnosed member was the main source of disturbance in the other members. While the child must always be seen in relation to his family, school and social setting, *it must never be forgotten that the diagnosis of the child is made in the child*. The presence of family distress, maternal anxiety and all the problems of disorganized families is no excuse for failure to examine the child as a patient in his own right.

An example of *gross family disorganization* is seen in the case of the sociopathic or 'multi-problem' family which is characterized by recurrent marital tensions and family breakdown. They display shallowness and violence of feelings, unpredictable and inconsistent child care, to a degree which necessitates the use of social agencies, or institutional care. These families have poor work records and reveal personality disorders and past deprivations within the parents; they are aware of their disability, resent their inadequacy, and are suspicious. They feel persecuted and are unable to trust; this makes any therapeutic approach difficult.

SOCIAL AND CULTURAL FACTORS

Different communities and cultures have different expectations, values and tolerance of children's behaviour and symptoms. The significance of children's behaviour may vary with social class, e.g. the professional family may see problems in their children that would not be seen by the family of an unskilled worker.

In different cultures, social and family structures vary, for example in extended families with their network of family figures, which make it difficult for external observers to assess and evaluate distress signals of children. Many social values, traditions and group behaviours are changing rapidly. In particular, social mobility involving geographic, economic, financial or social change imposes stress on the family and the development of children is influenced by community urbanization and geographic distance.

It is important to understand the cultural, ethnic values and family structure of migrant families and in particular how the parents perceive the child and interpret his symptoms. Due to language, cultural factors and factors related to migration, special training of professional workers is needed.

Factors commonly associated with poverty are related to one another and often perpetuate themselves into a cycle of poor physical and mental health, low income, chronic unemployment or unemployment, low education attainment, a cultural pattern of poverty and large families or broken families.

Changing family structure, marital breakdown, single parent families, parental vocation and employment opportunities, and the development of child care techniques, are current issues which need evaluation.

The maltreatment syndrome, describing children who are maltreated, presents as a problem of a breakdown of parenting, usually mothering, and is invariably associated with the parent's own early life experiences. The clinical problem, however, includes features of the child, parental health, the marital and family situation, current situational stresses and the reactions of society itself which may lead to social and even legal intervention.

In defining the physical, intellectual, emotional and social development of the child within the family and society, the child psychiatrist must develop techniques to define vulnerabilities and assets in the child, as well as the risk factors in the child's environment and their changing relevancy.

28

CHILDHOOD DISORDERS

The diagnosis of health and disorder in childhood should be made on positive grounds, recognizing that there are widely varying developmental norms in physical, intellectual, emotional and social growth. Children show the whole range of organic and functional psychiatric illnesses but also have special syndromes related to development such as minimal cerebral dysfunction.

The child must be viewed in the *framework of development* and not as a 'little adult'. Gross psychiatric disorders do not present the adult clinical pictures as seen in manic depressive illness and paranoid schizophrenia. Behaviour in children which is appropriate at certain stages of development may persist as a normal maturational lag, or where it is no longer appropriate it may indicate distress, e.g. enuresis. Distress is expressed in behaviour, so that disturbances of feeding, sleeping, enuresis and encopresis should be viewed as both physical and emotional.

The fact that symptoms change or disappear does not necessarily mean that the patient has improved. For instance, for the child with a personality disorder who has enuresis, the cessation of enuresis may have little practical significance in the total clinical picture.

This shows the need of being aware of the child's *distress signals*. A child is seldom self-referred and his referral may reflect the anxiety of those referring him rather distress in the child himself. In the early years of child psychiatry, 'nuisance' symptoms were commonly referred, such as aggressive behaviour, enuresis, encopresis or school failure—problems which brought the child into conflict with the accepted norms of his society. Later, people realized that the child could suffer within himself without putting out appropriate cues which would lead to medical referral. The inhibited, frightened child who fails to achieve can be potentially sicker than the child who has more aggressive distress signals which attract attention.

Attempts are now made to view the child as a whole rather than to compile an extensive symptom list. Nevertheless, symptoms are stresses for the child and may produce further disorder.

CLASSIFICATION*

A useful clinical classification of childhood disorders is:

(1) Healthy response
(2) Situational reaction (reactive disorders)

* For this classification I am indebted to the Group for Advancement of Psychiatry, 'Psychopathological Disorders in Childhood: Theoretical Consideration and a Proposed Classification', in their *Report*, vol. 6, no. 62 (June 1966).

(3) Developmental deviations
(4) Psychoneurotic disorders
(5) Personality disorders
(6) Psychotic disorders
(7) Psychophysiological disorders
(8) Brain syndromes
(9) Mental retardation

These conditions are not mutually exclusive. A child can occupy more than one category, and can move in the course of development from one to another.

HEALTHY RESPONSE

At certain stages in the child's development it is appropriate to show signs of anxiety. They are adaptive responses, but become problems when handled inappropriately. Examples are, the so-called eight months anxiety or stranger anxiety of the child; the separation anxiety of the young pre-school child; compulsive or ritualistic behaviour of the school-age child and the identity crisis of the adolescent. The important point here is that they are *stage appropriate* or *'phase specific' and their absence may be pathological.*

Reaction to a temporary situational crisis can also be regarded as a healthy response, such as the changes seen in a child following bereavement. He shows apathy, moodiness, refusal of food and other signs of distress, followed by attempts to work through his loss.

SITUATIONAL REACTIONS (REACTIVE DISORDERS)

Situational reactions (reactive disorders) occur when the behaviour or symptoms of the child are of a pathological degree and are related to an event or events or situations.

These are the common disorders of children who may suffer from stresses ranging from management problems, disturbed family relationships, school and social pressures to grosser stresses involving separation, bereavement, family disruptions, physical illness and other events. Children vary remarkably in their vulnerability to stress and it is not necessarily the *severity* of the stress which is the important fact, but the *signficance* of the stress in the light of their endowment and their past experience. Reactions to stress may be relatively appropriate or *adaptive*, e.g. aggressive behaviour or running away from danger. They may be *maladaptive* where the child under stress shows symptoms related to previous difficulties, e.g. wetting, soiling, or speech disturbance.

Infants and pre-school children are more sensitive to environmental stress and have not developed the internal defences of later years. Thus the child's choice of symptoms may give a good indication, not only of his current problems but also of difficulties experienced in his previous management. Sometimes the child's symptoms are part of family patterns of stress, where he repeats or imitates reactions of other members of the family.

173

DEVELOPMENTAL DEVIATIONS

As mentioned earlier there are wide norms for the common developmental stages, e.g. walking, speech and toilet-training, but some children seem to show innate difficulties in certain areas. Deviations may be single or multiple: they may be due to delayed maturation or congenital factors; they may even represent minimal damage in the early months or years for which the child can compensate later. Some deviations may be lifelong.

The following special areas should be considered:
(1) Motor development (including co-ordination and laterality)
(2) Sensory development
(3) Perceptual development (involving all sensory modalities)
(4) Speech development (involving articulation, receptive and expressive speech and language development)
(5) Cognitive development—delays in development of logical symbolic and abstract thinking, memory, reasoning and judgment make educational adjustment difficult.

Current research shows how much environmental factors influence the development or perpetuation of these developmental deviations, e.g. the role of speech stimulation in delayed language development.

PSYCHONEUROTIC DISORDERS

The neurotic process may begin in the early years but it is in the school years that neurotic disorders become clinically discernible. The child develops *defences* to control his sexual and aggressive drives. Impulses are repressed and later sublimated into socially acceptable channels. The core of the psychoneurotic disorder is the inner anxiety aroused by the child's conflicts which become internalized by repression. In children neurotic conflicts can be resolved by maturation, or become internalized and assume different clinical expressions. For example, separation anxieties unresolved in the pre-school years may lead to anxiety, phobic and depressive reactions when the child cannot cope later with the threat of separation—real or symbolic.

Each neurotic symptom is a compromise between the underlying wish or fear, the anxiety aroused and the defences against it. Clinically the traditional forms of neuroses are:
(1) The anxiety state
(2) Conversion reaction
(3) Dissociative reaction
(4) Obsessive-compulsive reaction
(5) Depressive reaction.

It is not intended to detail neurotic symptomatology again (see chapter 10) but these headings draw attention to clinical problems peculiar to children.

Anxiety which is undefended is experienced psychologically and physically as a typical anxiety reaction. It may be *displaced* on to some symbolic object or situation as in the phobic reaction.

It may be *converted* into various somatic symptoms as in conversion reaction; or it may *overwhelm* the individual and cause aimless activity or 'freezing', as in dissociative reactions. It may be *transposed* by means of various repetitions and reactions as in obsessive-compulsive reactions; and, finally, it *may allay itself by self-depreciation* as in the depressive reaction.*

(1) *Anxiety State*

Anxiety *symptoms* can be acute or chronic or phobic. The former are often precipitated by an illness, an operation or examinations and has the somatic and psychological symptoms described elsewhere. The chronically anxious child appears inhibited and fearful. Such children may be hypochondriacal and complain of ill health and inadequacy. Here family illness problems are important. Phobic symptoms commonly refer to animals, dirt, disease, high places or school.

(2) *Conversion Reaction*

'Conversion' is a *psychopathological concept* that implies a process of transforming anxiety into a dysfunction of bodily structures supplied by the voluntary portion of the nervous system involving the striate musculature and the somato-sensory apparatus.

Common conversion symptoms include disorders of function, such as motor (seen in paralysis and tics), sensory (blindness and deafness), speech (aphonia), hyperventilation, urinary (enuresis), abdominal pain and headache.

The diagnosis is made on positive grounds and not by exclusion. The clinical examination should study the whole patient: 'you examine the child to include the physical factors, not exclude them'.

Psychologically, the symptoms express the conflict symbolically, meet the child's immediate need and are the source of secondary gain. Conversion reactions most frequently appear in the 10- to 14-year-old girl.

The perpetuation of conversion reactions is strongly influenced by their management. The attitudes of parents and doctors are important as they may focus on the symptom and provide secondary gains.

(3) *Dissociative Reactions*

Here the child shows a gross temporary disorganization of personality, where overwhelming anxiety leads to apparently aimless behaviour, with amnesia, fugue states, depersonalization and disorders of consciousness, such as twilight states and stupor. These states are uncommon, are usually acute and monosymptomatic. The diagnosis is important: they should not be confused with psychotic or organic states which can produce apparently similar features.

* James Anthony, 'Psychoneurotic Disorders' in A. M. Freedman and H. I. Kaplan, *Comprehensive Textbook of Psychiatry*. Williams & Wilkins (Baltimore, 1967).

(4) Obsessive-Compulsive Reaction

The anxieties aroused by unconscious conflicts are counteracted by the occurrence of thoughts (obsessions) or impulses to act (compulsions) or mixtures of both. The child frequently recognizes his ideas or behaviour as being unreasonable, but is nevertheless compelled to repeat his rituals which often represent the opposite of his unconscious wish, e.g. excessive orderliness and washing compulsions overlie impulses to soil or mess.

Obsessions and compulsions of a minor kind begin early in life and may persist throughout childhood, such as the elaborate bedtime and feeding rituals of the toddler without which he cannot function comfortably.

Rituals may be associated with rigid routines on the part of compulsive parents who may foster the behaviour until it becomes too extreme for the child.

The onset of obsessional illness is usually in the school-age period, with a peak at nine years. Children who develop obsessional neuroses usually show previous evidence of anxiety, inhibitions, obsessiveness and shyness. Sometimes 'leakage symptoms' occur, e.g. the 'perfect child' with an obsessional personality whose encopresis reveals his conflict.

(5) Depressive Reaction

Depression in children and adolescents was originally thought to be uncommon. The thought of children feeling unhappy, worthless and hopeless—like the idea of children having sexual fantasies—was hard for adults to accept. The occurrence of suicide attempts in children can surprise doctors unaware of the problem.

In the early years the child is dependent on the 'object' world. Following 'object loss', he may show all the features of depression such as sadness, withdrawal, lack of interest, apparent retardation, regression, sleep disorder, restlessness, irritability and bodily concern. His behaviour may represent efforts to compensate for his loss and his dependence on the outside world is seen in clinging, demanding and hyperactive behaviour.

In the older child, response to object loss again depends on his level of development. The child with psychoneurotic disorder has internalized his conflicts. He is concerned with *fears of loss* and is caught in a love-hate relationship to his parents and other loved ones. His conflict is related to guilt about his angry feelings and his conflict anxiety is seen in feelings of unworthiness, sullenness and a sense of helplessness and of being abandoned.

Clinical features include sadness, weeping bouts, fears of death for himself and his parents, irritability, somatic complaints, loss of appetite and energy, sleep disturbance, difficult school adjustment, oscillation between clinging to and being hostile to his parents and self-depreciation.

Instead of depression, behaviour may occur which can be regarded as depressive equivalents. These include running away, accident proneness, boredom, restlessness and aggressive behaviour, which on investigation prove to be attempts to fend off feelings of depression, isolation, loneliness and emptiness. Suicidal thoughts may occur; suicide attempts may take place and suicide itself is not unknown. It should be remembered that, as in adults, depression associated with anxiety is a common accompaniment of organic diseases in childhood.

PERSONALITY DISORDERS

It is not customary to talk of personality disorders until later child-hood, when 'chronic or fixed pathological trends or traits have become ingrained in the personality structure'. Undoubtedly they exist earlier but developmental variations and stress reactions make the clinical picture less definite. Maturation and developmental spurts, more satisfactory environmental stimulation and opportunity for physical, intellectual, emotional and social experiences can all help the younger child to make a more favourable adjustment.

It is possible to form clinical categories of *predominant* traits in children which are present to a pathological degree. Two common examples are:

(1) *Isolated Personality*

This term refers to children who are distant, detached, cold and withdrawn in relationship to their family and friends. They are isolated, seclusive, unable to compete or to express healthy aggressive impulses. On occasions they show unpredictable outbursts of bizarre and aggressive impulses. They may achieve in certain areas, such as at school; they may also have a rich fantasy life, and be preoccupied with their own thoughts and ideas. It is unjustifiable to label them with terms such as 'pre-schizophrenic' or 'latent schizophrenic' and hence the description term 'isolated'.

(2) *Tension Discharge Disorders*

Children in this category have the most marked impact on family and society. The term is often used synonymously with *sociopathic personality*. These children show persistent discharge of sexual and aggressive feelings in conflict with society's norms, rather than repressing or inhibiting their impulses, or developing other symptoms. Terms such as *anti-social personality, psychopathic personality, impulsive character, affectionless character, acting out personality, neurotic character disorder, primary behaviour disorder, conduct disorder, delinquent character* have all been used at different times. The term 'tension discharge' pinpoints a central core of pathology without implicating concepts of permanence, aetiology, moral values and social norms.

These children show shallow relationships with adults and peers, low frustration tolerance, inadequate control of sexual and aggressive impulses which may be discharged without delay or inhibition and without regard for the consequences. Inner guilt is lacking and anxiety stems from the inability to control impulses and from the inevitable conflict between themselves and society. 'I want it, and I want it now', shows the inability to delay gratification. They are commonly presented to the clinic with *target symptoms* such as:

(1) Hyperactivity and aggressive behaviour

(2) Rages, emotionability, impulsiveness

(3) Immature speech, dyslalia, thumb-sucking, enuresis and other developmental delays

(4) School failure, academic and social

(5) Delinquent behaviour, e.g. arson, vandalism.

There is generally an early history of emotional deprivation from infancy and early childhood with frequent and prolonged separations, parental deaths or marital breakdowns. In developmental terms these children have been unable to establish trusting, satisfying and gratifying relationships. Consequently they are unable to move up the developmental scale and early forms of infantile gratifications persist. The normal child, who receives assurances that his parents are there and love him, can feel secure; he can postpone gratification and move on to more mature personality functioning. Disturbed behaviour often can be related to the parents' own psychopathology, the child acting out his parents' drives and wishes.

In these children it is not uncommon to find abnormal non-specific E.E.G. dysrhythmias without evidence of epilepsy, a finding which may represent delayed maturation.

The diagnosis must be made on a total evaluation of the child and his environment and not on target symptoms, however gross. Often a mutually destructive conflict between the child and his world has started and perpetuated a vicious circle.

The prognosis depends on many factors, but maturation continues throughout life; the number who persist with anti-social behaviour may be relatively few.

PSYCHOTIC DISORDERS

Childhood psychoses represent a severe disruption of personality functioning which may severely retard and distort personality development. They are relatively rare but may occur at any age.

Although it is only in recent years that psychotic disorders in children have been recognized, today the conditions tend to be over-diagnosed. It is important to be very specific in diagnosis. There is considerable controversy concerning the relationship of the various childhood psychoses to adult schizophrenia.

These severely disturbed children can be recognized by considering the following nine diagnostic points, keeping developmental variations in mind:

(1) There is gross and sustained impairment of emotional relationships.

(2) The child is apparently unaware of his own personal identity (compared with children of the same age).

(3) He is pathologically preoccupied with particular objects.

(4) He has sustained resistance to change in the environment and he strives to maintain or restore sameness.

(5) He has abnormal perceptual experiences as indicated by excessive, diminished or unpredictable response to sensory stimuli: for example, visual and auditory avoidance.

(6) In many cases he may show acute, excessive and seemingly illogical anxiety.

(7) He may have lost the ability to speak, or never acquired it, or he may have failed to develop it to a level appropriate to his age.

(8) His mobility patterns are distorted, e.g. hyperkinesis, immobility and bizarre postures.

(9) He has a background of serious retardation in which islets of normal or exceptional intellectual function or skill may appear.

Early Infantile Autism

In 1943 Kanner described eleven cases. By 1951 over 700 cases had been described in the literature. The pathognomic features of the disorder are:

(1) The child cannot relate himself in the ordinary way to people and situations from the beginning of life.

(2) He has an obsessive desire to maintain constancy of the environment.

(3) He displays marked anxiety if this constancy is threatened.

(4) He indulges in repetitive behaviour and is preoccupied with objects in a ritualistic and compulsive way.

(5) He does not use language for the purpose of communication.

Because of the early onset of the condition when interpersonal relationships are being established, there is marked uneven development with impairment of functions related to social behaviour, e.g. speech, though other areas of development may be normal.

In Kanner's syndrome, investigations revealed no known pathological cause. Intelligence was thought to be average and if the child did not develop speech before the age of five the prognosis was considered to be unfavourable. Parents of these children were described as cold, detached, obsessive and objective.

It is now realized that autistic behaviour is at times a normal developmental phenomenon. There may be mild autistic reactions to stress with complete or incomplete recovery. The condition occurs throughout all ranges of intelligence and may be associated with many pathological factors, e.g. known brain damage, deafness, phenylketonuria, mental retardation, epilepsy, visual, hearing and other neurological defects. Because of the varying conditions where this behaviour can be exhibited, some workers prefer the term 'autistic reaction' and the term 'early infantile autism' is reserved for those classical cases described by Kanner where no known pathology exists.

In such cases of early infantile autism two hypotheses have been suggested concerning possible aetiology: (1) that these children have a basic inability to integrate visual and auditory experiences into meaningful patterns; (2) that there is some dysfunction of the reticular activating system. There is insufficient evidence to favour either of these hypotheses.

All children presenting with autistic behaviour demand a full comprehensive diagnosis. A possible pathological cause may be the child's intellectual apparatus; particular attention should be paid to visual, auditory, perceptual and kinesthetic functions. The nature of the stresses which the child and the parents have experienced should be investigated. Professional workers are aware of the intense primitive emotional conflicts within these children which prevent them reaching out to the world. Their primitive defences of denial, isolation and withdrawal reflect their fear of the external world and their internalization of feelings of persecution.

Likewise workers are impressed with the intensity of the emotional problems of parents in relationship to the child. When they are offered therapeutic help, the stereotyped view of their child ('he is autistic', 'he is born different') tends to disappear and the conflict and problems of the early transaction between parent and child unfold.

However, environmental factors should not be viewed aetiologically, which would produce guilt, denial, hostility and intellectualization by adults, but rather as a necessary step in diagnosis and therapeutic understanding. Undoubtedly there are multiple determinants, varying manifestations of severity, and different outcomes. Some children become adult schizophrenics; others show a severe psychosis without developing the symptoms and signs that characterize schizophrenia.

In the psychoses of later childhood many workers prefer the term schizophreniform, implying that, though many of the clinical features are suggestive of schizophrenia, they do not reproduce features of the adult form nor do these children necessarily develop schizophrenia later.

Other forms of psychosis are seen in early childhood.

PSYCHOPHYSIOLOGIC DISORDERS

This term refers to disorders of organs inervated by the autonomic or involuntary parts of the central nervous system in which physical and psychological factors are important aetiologically (see chapter 14).

The child's condition is less static than the adult's because of his physical and psychological development; his distress signals, if recognized, are more obvious and his immaturity is an accepted and obvious feature of his behaviour. Therefore the child's dependent needs are usually met by his environment; in the adult, dependency needs may not be met or perhaps they are not even recognized by the adult himself. The immaturity of the child is associated with more flexibility and plasticity, whereas the adult has become more fixed and stereotyped in his response to stress. The child's immaturity permits the possibility of more avenues for discharge which, while partly decided by constitutional factors and also the specific nature of the stress, can still be strongly influenced by environmental factors, because the basis of the child's reaction is to achieve adaptive balance with his environment.

There is a constant interplay between genetic, constitutional and environmental experiences and these factors should not be ignored in any child. The child's management and handling in his environment may well decide the patterns of his responses to stress.

Bronchial Asthma

For purposes of illustration one common and important condition, bronchial asthma, will be described in detail.

Incidence and Prevalence

Most studies of asthmatic children have been made on selected populations, usually hospital or clinic populations, who have not remitted or responded to early treatment.

Wheezing attacks are common in young children and the relationship of asthma to wheezy bronchitis is not clear. Epidemiological findings suggest that children with wheezy bronchitis and asthma do belong to the same population with the same underlying basic disorders and that there is a wide spectrum in the aspects of the history of the disorder. It is estimated that up to 20% of all children have wheezed at some stage by the age of ten years, but the majority have ceased having asthma by that age and those children who persist into chronic persistent asthma form a very small subgroup in the region of 0·2%.

Aetiological factors include:
(1) Constitutional factors
(2) Allergic factors
(3) Infection
(4) Emotional factors.

While all of these factors may be important at different stages, the mere presence of one of them may not be a significant factor in the child's total clinical state. The constitutional factor is the *necessary* condition for the development of asthma; allergic, infective and emotional factors all contribute in varying degrees so that the threshold is reached for the asthmatic attack.

Psychological factors

Asthma affects children in all ranges of intelligence and all types of personality. Emotional factors in asthma have long been recognized and recent research suggests some constellation common to all asthmatic children. Those which precipitate attacks are non-specific; anxiety, anger or excitement may precipitate an attack under circumstances which affect a particular child, e.g. entry to school, family stresses. Some attacks are produced by frightening thoughts or fears: children with nocturnal asthma frequently describe frightening dreams wakening them and precipitating an attack.

In cases referred for psychiatric consultation children commonly describe an attack as including feelings of suffocation, helplessness, strangling, being crushed and fears of dying; such descriptions when elaborate could indicate additional neurotic components in the condition. The attack produces an enforced dependence and fear of separation from the mother who the child nevertheless realizes is helpless to deal with his distress. This initial awareness leads to a high level of maternal anxiety, fear of death and future attacks and a reaction of overprotection and dependence. The mother-child relationship becomes characterized by separation anxiety, anxious dependence leading to regressive behaviour in the child and defence against this. The mother may fear this, and over-react, and this may lead to further anxiety. The child may become unable to express his feelings healthily, and handle situations by denial, inhibition or poor control.

There may then develop a marked relationship between the mother's emotional state and the child's asthma: depression and anxiety in the mother is related to asthma or disturbed behaviour which heightens the mother's anxiety and leads to further asthma in the child and further emotional tension in the mother. Precipitating factors may increase as both the asthma and its effects tend to diminish the child's ability to cope with stresses (e.g. school), further heightening his anxieties. Secondary gains may become apparent, sometimes culminating in the child's ability to produce an attack consciously as an avoidance mechanism. At this stage the parents who have reacted to the child's problem with such emotions as anxiety, fear, denial and guilt, may perceive it as manipulative. Management may then alternate between ignoring the asthma and overprotection.

The condition is commonly perpetuated by often unreal aetiological importance being given to family history and genetic background; this produces a sense of uncertainty. Pathogens held responsible for attacks (e.g. pollen, food, climate, housing, excitement, parties) cause the parents to surround the child with unreal precautions; he perceives the world as dangerous and this increases his anxiety. Structural damage which restricts his pulmonary function adds a further physical handicap.

In these cases it is common for asthma to cease when a child is admitted to hospital and recur when he returns home. When his mother visits he may cry and wheeze; because of this it is common to use the hospital and separation from home as a form of treatment. This can abort the attack with appropriate medical care and the process of separation, but there are dangers inherent in the situation, because it will further diminish the child's confidence and trust in his parents and increase mutual awareness that asthma occurs at home because of the mother-child interaction. The return home will often increase the emotional problem and produce more dependence on the hospital thus perpetuating the vicious circle. On the other hand the family's situation and the child's physical health may be such that they demand these measures in any case. Experience in residential treatment settings for asthmatic children has emphasized to all workers the necessity for a psychotherapeutic approach to the child and his family.

BRAIN SYNDROMES

These are disorders caused by impairment of brain function by maldevelopment, structural damage or malfunction without apparent structural change.

Organic brain syndromes in children show certain features which are different to the adult clinical picture:

(1) They are more able to 'compensate' for brain damage.

(2) The more recently acquired functions are most vulnerable so that *regression* is a marked clinical feature.

(3) The organic insult may distort developmental patterns so that it is difficult to judge the severity of the lesion from the presenting symptoms.

(4) The family's ability to understand and meet the child's needs is important in permitting the child to adjust to his defect.

A comprehensive diagnostic assessment is needed in each child; particular attention should be paid to motor functions, co-ordination, ataxia, tremors, vision, hearing, perception, language, development, memory and reasoning. Epilepsy must be considered.

Accurate observations are important for diagnosis and management.

Emotionally the child reacts to his condition within the limits of his personality resources (mediated by his family and social management). Anxieties relating to the damage itself, his self-awareness and ability to cope may prevent healthy recovery. Animistic thinking and concepts of causality may make him feel he was attacked, hurt, or damaged as a punishment. In fact, the whole range of psychiatric disorders may be seen as a secondary part of the picture, e.g. neurotic, psychotic or behavioural disturbances.

Acute brain syndromes are characterized by delirium, confusion, impairment of orientation, discrimination, learning and memory, as well as lability of affect. Causes include systemic infections, intracranial infection, intoxications due to drugs or poisons, trauma, and convulsive, circulatory and metabolic disturbances.

Sub-clinical delirium is often missed and is characterized by fluctuations of levels of attention, awareness, anxiety, mild stupor and withdrawal.

Chronic brain syndromes: where there is permanent impairment, the child shows the same nuclear symptoms, and signs of cognitive and emotional disturbance. Perseveration, slowness, poverty of thought, difficulty in maintaining attention and vulnerability to disorientation, are the diagnostic symptoms but emotional difficulties are often the *presenting* symptom.

Management involves not only a comprehensive evaluation of the child, but also that of his family and school. It is remarkable that when these children's needs are understood and met by appropriate measures (e.g. educational and school adjustment and relief of inappropriate stress) his anxiety is lessened favourably; with further development and maturation remarkable compensation can occur.

The Concept of Minimal Cerebral Dysfunction

A child handicapped by major disabilities is described in terms of the dominant defect, e.g. motor defect, cerebral palsy, blind or deaf. To explain presenting features with *minimal* handicaps, many terms have been used over the years implicating brain injury, e.g. the brain-damaged child. Such terms imply an aetiology which can rarely be demonstrated and usually there is no pathological evidence of actual cerebral damage. Further, cerebral injury can exist without accompanying clinical pictures. Sometimes the *child is labelled* by the dominant presenting symptom e.g. the 'hyperkinetic child', a term which ignores his other attributes and may imply a uniform and permanent clinical picture.

The most recent term to define this problem is *minimal cerebral dysfunction* which indicates the minimal nature of the defects and their neurological component. Although the term dysfunction recognizes the functional component, this definition permits aetiologies ranging from genetic variations, biochemical irregularities, perinatal brain insults, other illness; they may arise from unknown causes or from injuries sustained during the years which are critical for the development and maturation of the central nervous system. The definition also allows for the possibility that early severe deprivation could result in central nervous system alterations which may be permanent. Characteristic of this syndrome are:

(1) Hyperactivity
(2) Perceptual and motor impairment
(3) Emotional lability

(4) General co-ordination defects
(5) Disorders of attention (short attention span, distractibility)
(6) Impulsiveness
(7) Disorders of memory and thinking
(8) Specific learning disabilities (reading, writing, spelling, arithmetic)
(9) Disorders of speech and hearing
(10) Equivocal neurological signs and electro-encephalographic irregularities.

These clinical characteristics are target symptoms. Each area of the child's 'apparatus' must be assessed to detect the presence of minimal handicaps and assess their impact on the child's functioning. The child is often able to cope behaviourally, but is prone to anxiety, and attainment of control is difficult. He tends to disorganize or become disinhibited under stress, he becomes fatigued quickly and at times shows perseveration. These handicaps may impair his attention-concentration span, lower his tolerance for frustration and impair his interest in task orientation. In clinical practice, there may be marked variance between the degree of handicap and the child's ability to adapt behaviourally due to strengths which should be looked for and *used*.

Developmental Aspects

Many cases of minimal cerebral dysfunction may be regarded as maturational defects where the rate of development in various areas is uneven; each deficit leads to compensatory mechanisms, e.g. a clumsy child may prefer talking and reading. These deviations, however, are *necessary* conditions, limiting opportunities for learning. Sufficient conditions lie in the *learning conditions* and *models* which have been offered to the child. The child may need appropriate stimulation at the so-called period of readiness.

Epidemiological studies relating to social class, and other studies relating to deprivation and stress, indicate the importance of environmental influences. Developmental deviations in the child impose stress on the mother-child relationship which is more likely to be disturbed if the child is minimally handicapped. The child with specific defects has difficulties in responding, and also imposes a frustration on himself which affects the mother-child bond.

It is important to assess the parents' capacity to cope with this vulnerable child and their ability to understand and recognize his difficulties. Such a disturbance can make the child a focus of the parents' anxieties; these may be concerned with particular functions in the child, e.g. speech or hyperactivity, which will further increase his difficulties. The *presenting focus* of a child with such difficulties is *often highly influenced by parental choice*. There are now available well-controlled studies indicating that there is no uniform minimal cerebral dysfunction behavioural clinical syndrome, and no one pattern of behavioural dysfunction.

MENTAL RETARDATION

Through the ages most cultures and societies have recognized the severely retarded individual. Mental retardation itself is a symptom with many causes and the patient's individual behaviour is influenced by genetic, medical, psychological and social factors.

Classifications

Early studies suggested that a separation could be made into:

(1) A *subcultural type* which was regarded as a genetic variation within a community, and an extreme end of the normal range of mental abilities. This was the larger group.

(2) *Pathological types*, where there were known physical causes.

However, more recent work has drawn attention to the importance of *emotional* and *social* factors in most retarded children, as well as biological factors which affect brain function.

Modern classification now refers to:

(1) A biological group with known physical causes.

(2) An environmental group with psychological, social and cultural factors, including deprivation, poor nutrition, inadequate emotional and intellectual stimulation in economically, educationally and socially deprived families and relatively adverse cultural backgrounds.

(3) An intermediate group where both biological and environmental factors operate.

In the most common mild type of mental retardation, physical causes must be looked for, though usually they will not be found.

The Role of Heredity

Most parents of mentally retarded children are not retarded. In a small number of patients genetic defects are found, Down's syndrome being the most frequent.

Prevalence

Estimates and criteria vary between countries. In general, intelligence tests indicate that $1-4\%$ of school-age children are mentally retarded. The vast majority of these (75%) are mildly retarded and a small number (0.3%) are severely retarded. After school age there is an abrupt drop—most blend into the general population.

Aetiology

In all patients three factors should be assessed. These are:

(1) Pathological
(2) Psychological
(3) Social.

A full clinical understanding of the whole problem and particularly the management of the child and family cannot be made without study of (2) and (3).

Pathological factors may be classified:

(1) Infections: antenatal and perinatal, e.g. rubella, meningitis, encephalitis, cytomegalic inclusive body disease, toxoplasmosis

(2) Intoxication: severe prolonged toxaemia of pregnancy, bilirubin encephalopathy, lead and other poisons

(3) Trauma, e.g. birth injury, anoxia, postnatal injury

(4) Disorders of metabolism: e.g. phenylketonuria, cretinism, hypoglycaemia, galactosaemia, cerebral lipoidosis

(5) Tumours, e.g. tuberosclerosis, neurofibromatosis

(6) Unknown prenatal influences, e.g. Down's, Klinefelter's syndromes, congenital cerebral defects.

(7) Unknown causes without physical signs, e.g. cultural-familial mental retardation, environmental deprivation—the largest group.

In each instance the presence or absence of genetic factors, cranial anomalies, special sense and perceptual disorders, epilepsy, cerebral palsy and psychiatric disorders need to be noted. The student is referred to main textbooks for accounts of individual conditions.

Two conditions can be treated directly.

(1) *Phenylketonuria*

This defect is one of the many rare recently discovered biochemical defects which accounts for 2–3% of severely retarded children. The defects are inherited as a recessive gene with a risk of 1 in 4 that other children in these families will be affected; phenylketonuria is the most common. There is a biochemical enzyme defect (incidence 1 per 10,000) where phenylalanine (an essential amino acid) cannot be metabolized, resulting in an accumulation of phenylalanine and related substances with spill into the urine. This can be detected at 4–6 weeks using ferric chloride or phenistix test (green reaction). Accumulation of these substances impairs cerebral metabolism and consequent mental development; if untreated the child will be mentally retarded. These children are frequently fair-haired, subject to convulsions from infancy, and often have eczema. Dietary treatment should be started as soon as possible. For this reason the Guthrie blood test is now widely used. Where there is a known family history, serum phenylalanine and urinary chromatography should be carried out.

(2) *Cretinism*

There is persistent physiological jaundice immediately after birth, a reluctance to feed, and constipation. There is a characteristic facial appearance, coldness of the skin and paucity of movements. Bone age is retarded. Treatment with thyroxine needs to be started early.

Down's syndrome (Mongolism) is one of the few conditions which can be diagnosed at birth with which mental retardation to some significant degree is invariably associated. The chromosomal complement is usually increased from 46 to 47 due to trisomy of 21. The chance of another mongol is 1–100. In a rare form there are 46 chromosomes with trisomy of 21 with translocation of the third chromosome to one member of another pair. Such an abnormality, if present, may occur with half of later children. Advice to the parents will therefore depend upon the chromosomal abnormality present. The child should be carefully examined for associated congenital defects.

Examination

(1) *Physical*

A careful physical examination should be carried out, paying particular attention to the following:

(1) Physical characteristics
(2) Vision and hearing; the child's ability to respond to sound and language should always be studied
(3) Presence of other congenital defects
(4) Abnormal neurological signs.

In infants the maximum head circumference just above the base of the nose must be measured so that the rate of increase may be measured. The optic fundii should be examined in all cases for optic atrophy, choriorentinitis and other abnormalities. Factors such as physical health, nutrition, sensory defects, pigmentation (P.K.U.) may help in diagnosis. The examiner should be aware of the possibilities of epilepsy in its various forms. Biochemical screening is mandatory.

(2) *Psychological and Behavioural*

It is stated that the retarded child is slow in all areas. Although he is able to relate to the examiner, his responses are often delayed and give a rapid clue to his level of intellectual development. However, in any examination it is important to note his motivation and interests, his ability to attend and comprehend the situation and to persevere with the task. These must be assessed in relation to the child's activities and interests and his emotional responses to success or failure. His level of understanding of the task may range from simple manipulative repetition to an ability to undertake the task in a similar situation appropriately, and later be able to generalize to other situations.

These factors will distinguish:

(1) the withdrawn or autistic child who is unable to relate
(2) the emotionally inhibited, frightened or aggressive child
(3) the distractible, restless child
(4) the child who perseverates and is unable to move on to new learning

(5) the child with poor control who readily becomes anxious and disorganized and responds to frustration with, e.g. tantrums.

In the older child more definite signs of anxiety may be seen with denial: for instance he may resort to inappropriate behaviour or fantasy.

Careful examination will nearly always reveal areas of strengths and weaknesses which indicate how the child can best be helped and where he may need specific treatment. For this reason, the child should be carefully screened for defects of his apparatus as described earlier, e.g. motor, vision, hearing, perception, language and cognitive disorders. Conditions such as cerebral palsy may be overlooked in infancy because spasticity may not develop until later in the first year of life.

The *reality conditions of the examination* should always be borne in mind. For instance the examination may take place in a crowded room, or when the child is tired, hungry or separated from his mother. It is most important to observe evidence of learning *within* the clinical interview and then look for evidence of this learning in later interviews. The initial interview gives evidence of the child's current level of functioning. Progress over a period of time is important to assess improvement (through learning or maturation) or deterioration.

(3) *Psychological Techniques*

The use of developmental scales as screening devices is helpful. However, a comprehensive psychological assessment should be carried out by trained psychologists whose examination may include the use of various standardized techniques. Psychological testing at first emphasized intellectual aspects of behaviour with an undue reliance on 'intelligence tests'. I.Q.s were often used as a global score, sometimes unintentionally implying permanence. Since then psychological examinations have emphasized qualitative aspects of the child's behaviour and noted modifiable emotional and social factors. Psychologists take into account in their evaluation technical problems such as which tests are used, what they measure, their validity and reliability and also the problems of administering them to retarded children with varied social experiences.

Repeated psychological examinations are important because they provide standardized measures of the child's present status relating him to other children of similar age.

(4) *Social Diagnosis*

The socially deprived child may commonly show evidence of malnutrition, under-stimulation and lack of appropriate care. The family may be unable to provide adequate social models for the child to learn from. Such children, because they lack social confidence, may show evidence of lack of self-care, may lack interest and motivation;

they may be unable to interact appropriately with others, and their behaviour is directed to their own needs and wishes. Such children fail on structured tasks, such as psychological tests.

Management

Management begins with the first interview and should continue in a planned way throughout the child's life, recognizing his needs at different ages. After a careful and comprehensive diagnosis of the child, appropriate treatment should be commenced for the small group of conditions where specific therapy is indicated, e.g. P.K.U., cretinism. The handicap of mental retardation imposes a stress on the child himself and the family and is a challenge to his society and the community.

The Family

The parents and family should be studied at the initial examination to assess the parents' personalities, their perception of the child and understanding of his difficulties, and their willingness and ability to cope with a handicapped child. Parents are usually aware that the child is delayed in his development; their anxiety and fear for his well-being may influence his development. For instance they may over-protect him; they may stimulate inappropriately because they expect too much or too little; they may be unable to offer appropriate learning situations and discipline.

The parents may attempt to find reasons for his difficulty; they may feel they have caused it themselves and that other people realize this. In their distress they may show evidence of depression and depend too much on specialists; or they may deny the child's difficulties, overtly hoping that he will be 'all right', or they may search further for unrealistic cures.

In some social settings there is considerable ignorance, superstition and fear, e.g. unrealistic fears that he will affect other children in the family, or if placed with other retarded children he will deteriorate, or if the neighbours know of him the family will be ostracized. For these reasons various manifestations of *over-protection* and *rejection* of the child may be evident.

The place of the child in the family may be important, e.g. there are special problems for the *only* child. The family's social position and economic situation (e.g. housing, opportunities for play) may limit possible therapeutic programmes but the family's willingness and ability to receive help are more important. Some families will react to the stress of having a retarded child by becoming more disrupted while others will become more closely united. The handicapped child may have special meaning for one parent and may serve as a focus for mutual blame. It is specially difficult for the father to adjust to the realization that his child is handicapped; the effect may be that the mother becomes more closely bound to the child and the father moves away into activities at work or outside interests.

The findings of the present examination should be conveyed to the parents at their own level so that they realize the difficulties of making a prognosis. Few conditions are obvious at birth and usually the diagnosis of retardation emerges during later development. It is essential that any necessary examination be carried out immediately, e.g. urine, X-ray of skull, etc., and that the condition be discussed with the parents; they must have a realistic appreciation of the relevance of the physical findings, and know how the child's needs can best be met. *It is never appropriate to 'wait and see'.* At each stage the mother should be helped with a positive programme to stimulate the child at his level. Advice should be practical and concrete.

The physician should always be receptive to the parents' fears and anxieties; reactions of anxiety, fear, guilt and, most important, depression should be handled sensitively. It is important to include both parents in early contact. The mother and family will need time to adjust emotionally; repeated interviews will be necessary before they are able to cope objectively. The initial impact may make the mother feel that she cannot cope and that the child is better off with specially trained people in an institution. The parents should be encouraged to love and care for their child, and helped to understand and manage him. Any decision to institutionalize the child must be made objectively; panic decisions made at the early stages may lead to considerable guilt and regret later. *The child's physical and emotional needs are usually best met within the family who can prepare him to attend appropriate day programmes*, e.g. special schools, groups, etc. Children who have benefited through the care of the family when young may later benefit from institutionalization.

Rarely the child may have to be put in hospital because of his gross congenital anomalies. During the hospitalization the mother can be helped emotionally and practically to learn the nature of his condition and how to relate to him.

At an appropriate time the nature of genetic factors should be discussed and the parents helped to face further pregnancies realistically. Some parents may need help at a practical level, and home visiting by professionally trained workers can be useful. In most countries it is difficult to provide adequate pre-school or nursery training for the retarded child because there are few facilities.

More recently techniques are being devised to facilitate diagnosis and planned treatment through the use of *groups* for retarded children, where they may be observed in a small group by a team of trained workers. In this setting it is possible to observe the child's level of development in relation to other children, his predominant methods of behaviour, his ways of communicating and his capacity to relate to other children and adults and to cope with various tasks. *Within the setting a child is encouraged to play and interact with other children.* His emotional behaviour can be studied and factors such as separation anxiety can be seen. Often apparatus defects, e.g. hearing, language and minor motor defects, may be more easily observed. When the child is observed over several sessions, the possibility of his attendance at school or day centre can be assessed. The group provides opportunities both for individual interviews with the mother and for her to meet other mothers whose children are handicapped. The use of group work with parents can be extremely valuable and rewarding, through the help of a professionally trained worker, e.g. psychiatrist, psychologist or social worker. The parents are encouraged to discuss problems relevant to the child and this gives them the opportunity for active, co-operative participation in and direction of their children's care. Mutual doubts and successful techniques in management can be shared with other parents. Feelings of resentment, hostility and blame may be directed at doctors, obstetricians, etc. and theurapeutic work by the parents' group may decisively help the parent and serve as a useful adjunct to individual work.

The Problem of Institutionalization

With certain types of handicapped children the question of admitting them to an institution will inevitably arise. Except where there are urgent considerations the decision should *not* be made at once, but ideally when the parents are able to view the problem more objectively. Formerly the trend towards permanent institutionalization together with the lack of appropriate facilities often made this decision extremely difficult for parents. Modern trends include short-term placements either to provide rest for the parents or during periods of family crisis.

Smaller residential units are now preferred and cottage-type facilities for these children are being planned. Studies have shown that the dangers of institutionalization are lessened when children live in small groups in an atmosphere resembling a family home, with practical aids to adjust to more normal home living, e.g. children with mild orthopaedic handicaps can be helped by splinting and walking machines. Two groups of factors will influence the decision to place the child in an institution:

(1) *Factors in the Child*

Three types of children may benefit from institutionalization:

(a) Children with severe handicaps (e.g. paralysis, incontinence) who cause difficulties in nursing.

(b) Severely retarded children who place too heavy a burden on the family.

(c) Children with disorders of behaviour (e.g. hyperactivity, destructiveness) who will need special treatment programmes.

(2) *Social Factors*

The commonest reasons for placing a child in an institution are social factors, such as family breakdown and inability to cope with the child's needs despite realistic practical help in the home setting. Where the child's behaviour produces anxieties and family tensions which cannot be reduced by a sympathetic and realistic therapeutic help, temporary placement permits those aspects to be handled more purposefully. It is most important for parents to know that their child will be cared for if they are sick or die.

The family whose child is being placed in an institution needs considerable help and counselling, which can be offered particularly when they visit the child.

Day Training Centres

Centres are available for children who are considered 'ineducable', i.e. unsuitable for admission to the normal schools or special schools for the mildly subnormal child. All children need a careful comprehensive assessment before admission and the psychologist's findings are most important. The child's ability to attend to tasks, his social behaviour, level of activity, etc. may influence the preference for day-centre management. This should not be thought of as a permanent placement but rather as a stage in the child's socialization and training. Some children may improve sufficiently to leave the day training centre and enter a school.

The Special Day School

Most educational departments have created special schools for mildly subnormal children. They provide special methods, modified curricula, specialized teachers and more teachers per child. Probably the large class is the single factor which most prevents satisfactory education of the subnormal. The duller the child, the more need he has of individual help. The special school is able to construct teaching programmes better adapted to the handicapped child's needs; these needs may vary considerably from child to child and within children during their development. The many handicaps which face retarded children, e.g. poor physique, lack of stamina, physical handicaps, perceptual problems, memory and other common difficulties, all need to be recognized and planned for. Difficulties in concentration, emotional adjustment, motivation and other factors can be handled by appropriate programmes. The child's social training is most important; special help such as psychotherapy, speech therapy, physiotherapy and remedial teaching should be available.

Vocational choice and guidance

Considerable anxiety is experienced by retarded children and their parents as the children approach adolescence. The problems of their future role in life, their ability to get a job amongst ordinary people or need for provision such as sheltered workshops are causes of anxiety. In some countries this aspect has been neglected until recently. The many years of specialized help suddenly ceased and the child's vocational and social handicap threw him back on to his family, the members of whom were now much older. Education departments now arrange careful vocational guidance and planned transition into a job, often using training workshops and other training devices as intermediate steps from the special schools.

The mentally retarded adolescent may have special problems beyond those encountered by other adolescents. Realization of his handicap may increase his inadequacy and resentment and he may be unable to gain full control of his sexual and aggressive feelings. Peer relationships, recreation and leisure activities are extremely important for him, and the formation of clubs and other group activities are extremely valuable.

Parent Groups

Parent-group associations may provide opportunities for parents not only to obtain help for family problems but, by mutual discussion, to relate to other families similarly placed and above all to improve the place of the retarded child through energetic social activities. This involves the education of the public, and parent groups may often help to arouse a more realistic appreciation of the problems of the retarded child and the urgent need for recognition and help. With realistic and purposive education a variety of voluntary groups can assist with different aspects of this complex problem.

29

PRINCIPLES OF MANAGEMENT

REFERRAL

The child will usually be brought to the psychiatrist because he is a problem to someone. The reason will depend on many factors, including the values, feelings and personalities of the parents, current fashions of society and ignorance of the normal variations in behaviour during development. The problem may be in the child or in the perception of the child by the environment; in either case, relationships of the child to his environment are disturbed. One therefore asks four basic questions: (1) who is the child? (2) who brought him? (3) why did they bring him? and (4) why did they bring him now?

THE SYMPTOMS

Children seldom refer themselves. The symptom is the presenting feature which has caused people to refer him. It may not be 'the problem' but it shows that there is a problem. The referral does not necessarily locate the difficulty or show its significance for the particular patient. Some symptoms are emphasized, others ignored. Some parents see no problem where other parents panic. Symptoms may have different meanings to both parents and child; they have different meanings in different social settings. For example, delinquency in a 'proper' household has a different significance to delinquency in a delinquent area of society.

DIAGNOSIS

Nosological clinical diagnoses in child psychiatry have been unsatisfactory when based on target symptoms, because these bear different connotations: enuresis is a physical sign; delinquency is a social concept; mental retardation is a behavioural symptom; cretinism refers to endocrine pathology. These tell little of the child, and in particular of their developmental significance. The psychopathological framework used in this chapter provides an understanding of the child. A symptom such as enuresis can be seen as an age-appropriate phenomenon in a young pre-school child under the heading, *healthy response*; as a symptom of a regressive nature in a *reactive disorder*; as a continuing feature of a *developmental deviation*; as part of a neurotic picture involving *conversion mechanisms*; or as one symptom in a *chronic personality disorder* or a *psychotic reaction* or *brain syndrome*.

To reach a diagnosis the processes which produce the child's present difficulties must be understood. Current environmental pressures interact with the child's internal forces (needs, conflicts, anxieties) to produce symptoms (dynamic diagnosis). Through clinical history and examination their *developmental* significance can be assessed (genetic diagnosis). Current findings can be evaluated in the *perspective* of the child's *development* and *life situation*. Assessment can frequently foresee spontaneous remission, deterioration and other outcomes.

Three areas of diagnosis should be studied:
(1) the child: individual pathology
(2) the family: family pathology
(3) social and cultural factors: social pathology.

CLINICAL EVALUATION

Many sources of information concerning the child and his family may be available spontaneously or on enquiry. However, it is in the clinical interview that the child and his caretaker present themselves and their problems. Diagnosis and therapy take place through the relationship with the physician.

The child and his family arrive at the office of the physician who notes which members attend, their behaviour and the presenting focus of concern. Different methods are used to make contact from an interview with the whole family or a brief family contact leading to individual interview with particular members of the family. In each case while the presenting anxieties of the parents are evaluated there is a cardinal rule: the diagnosis of the child is made in the child who, through his verbal and non-verbal behaviour, can alone provide his own history giving relevance to his past and present experiences. The aim is to establish a warm and trusting relationship with the child and to avoid creating difficulties which can occur if the child, particularly an older child, is not seen alone earlier. Some physicians prefer to see the parents first, sometimes by separate appointments so that the physician can focus on the child alone when he attends later. This can help the parents clarify their problems. However, the dangers (which usually outweigh the advantages) are (1) the child's reaction to this apparent collusion; (2) the bias created in the physician about this 'unseen' and as yet unknown patient; (3) the neglect of the most valuable observation of the parents and child together. In family interviews the style of the family, the relationships within it, and members' perceptions of each other can be observed. Work proceeds with the participation of all from the start.

(1) Relationship

The relationship of the child to the physician is influenced by the circumstances surrounding the interview and also by the previous life experiences of both participants. The child is usually brought by parents, or other caretakers; he may be ignorant, anxious, resentful, guilty or apprehensive about the purpose of the interview. He may be unsure of the physician, and suspect or distrust him: he may perceive him as an ally of parents or of a critical society. The deprived or dependent child, on the other hand, may seek help unrealistically. The physician, aware of this must also be sensitive to the child's methods of communication, and the level of his development and understanding; he must be prepared to 'tune into' whatever 'behavioural pseudopodia' the child puts out. He must learn the child's thoughts and feelings through work, play and fantasy, and be secure in his ability to cope with the child's often uncontrolled behaviour when driven by intense sexual and aggressive feelings. The child who demands physical contact, or who physically attacks or loses control or shows his greed, exposes the physician to primitive, undisguised, intense feelings, which are often regressive and infantile.

The physician should relate to the child's emotional experience, but be able to control his own reactions and use them to serve the child's needs and conflicts. Some common problems, for example, may be seen in:

(1) Separation anxiety—often reciprocated by the parent

(2) Silence—which may represent anxiety, anger, hostility, guilt, shame, or an attempt to control the interview

(3) Negativism—manifested often as conventional responses, or 'I don't know'; 'I forget'

(4) Aggressive, testing, provocative behaviour—often attacking objects in the room, the physician or even himself

(5) Sudden panics and anxiety attacks

(6) Overcontrol with rigid, stereotypic, guarded or obsessional behaviour.

All these apparent difficulties, however, are important clues. The child's characteristics are studied in the interview and such behavioural responses to the interviewer tell the story of his conflicts.

By the use of words and play, knowledge is built up concerning (1) the child's concept of himself, that is his sense of identity; (2) the child's perception of and feelings about his world, his parents, siblings and others; (3) the school, which includes his attitude to school work, peers, teachers and other authoritative figures, and finally (4) his perception of the larger world.

(2) The Child's Play as a Clinical Tool

Play is a natural activity of the child, commencing in infancy and continuing throughout development. In the clinical interview, play is a natural tool for expression and communication especially for the young child. It serves many purposes and tells much about the child's interests, skills, fantasies and fears, and depicts dramatically his inner emotional life. By observing the child playing one can easily assess developmental levels, become aware of his special skills and of defects, such as clumsiness, handedness, difficulties with perception or language.

In his play the child gives indications concerning his wishes, his perception of the world. In his fantasy, he can reveal his feelings, hopes, pleasures and difficulties. In his play he prepares for future functions and finds solutions to situations, providing him with pleasure and satisfaction. In play he creates his own reality so that he can do things not permitted in 'real life'. In technical terms, he takes leave of absence from reality and from the superego. A disturbed child will reflect his conflicts in play. The repetition in play of previous traumatic events enables him to deal again with painful situations; by actively reversing the roles, he actively masters painful events. Where the child's emotional intensity is greatest, there are in his play repetitive related themes which permit gradual assimilation of anxiety. The very disturbed child may be unable to play, or he may confuse reality with fantasy, or remain fixed, unable to find adaptive solutions. In the clinical interview, a disturbed child may use play as a defence rather than a shared activity with the physician, and so defend and isolate himself.

The physician should note that the child is writing the script and the physician is there to read the plot, act as auxiliary stage manager and help the child understand his anxieties and help him reach favourable solutions.

Understanding play is fundamental to understanding children clinically; it is not just childish behaviour obstructing the 'good stuff' of the interview. 'When I was a child, I spake as a child, I understood as a child, I thought as a child, but when I became a man I put away childish things': St Paul cogently shows the adult's initial difficulty in communicating with children.

Children respond to a trusting relationship with an adult who is concerned *for them*; when approached a child will talk of his difficulties. Questions appropriate to his level of development, should be framed to avoid the conventional response. Avoid an interchange like this: 'Do you like school?' 'All right.' 'How did you get on?' 'Not bad.' Encourage the child to tell what he feels is important. The use of drawings, stories, reading, writing, arithmetic and games can be helpful. While different interviews may have different goals, observation should provide the physician with varied information relating to the child. This should include observation of

(1) Physical functioning: his growth, general health, physical activity, skills and handicaps.

(2) Intellectual functioning: both the overall level and specific areas of cognitive function.

(3) Emotional functioning: whether his behaviour is appropriate to his age, his *relationship* to physician, parents, siblings and others; his

personality features, sense of identity; whether he sees himself and the people around him realistically; his level of anxiety; how he copes with stress; his motivation, his adaptability and his tolerance for frustration; his capacity to work and play.

(4) Social functioning: his social relationships and skills at home, and with other adults; his educational progress, academic skills, and relationships within the school; special interests such as his hobbies; his participation in and membership of groups, his social activities including antisocial or social behaviour.

(3) *The Use of Groups*

Much useful diagnostic information can be obtained by observing the child within a group and noting his relationships to peers and teachers: the nature of his activity, his social behaviour (leadership, passivity, isolation, aggression) and his ability to handle this more socially exacting situation. Anxious, fearful, aggressive children, or children with minimal handicaps can be identified and their frustrations understood.

(4) *Interviewing Parents*

The parents bring to the interview their concern for their child. Their observations of the child's behaviour may or may not be objective, but the parents, through their account, reflect their own feelings, fears, anxieties and guilt, and their defences against them.

In the course of the clinical history, where the parents are encouraged to talk freely, it is possible to examine the nature of their relationship to the child, how realistically they perceive him and what their reactions are to the child's behaviour at different developmental phases. It is important to see what the parents think is healthy or inappropriate, and how they react to the child.

In disturbed families, retrospective information about the early developmental history is commonly distorted, but it indicates the parents' perception of the child's developmental processes. The parents' account should be seen in the total context of the processes which interrelate and affect each other. To regard parents as the problem can only intensify, or even create, guilt, resentment and anger. It does not help the parents or the child.

The diagnostic interview includes consideration of current difficulties, a developmental history of the child within the context of the family's experiences and the presenting psychological mechanisms and defences. The presence of feelings such as guilt, anxiety, depression, anger, frustration, disappointment, shame, together with an understanding of the parent-child and family relationships determine the planning of treatment.

The relevance of emotional disturbance in the parents for the child must always be understood. Sometimes the child is in a 'conflict-free zone', not specially involved and therefore able to cope. Indeed a child is often able to help a parent's recovery from emotional distress.

Joint interviews and family interviews are useful techniques for diagnosis and, in certain cases, therapy. Some presenting symptoms in the child are dramatically significant in this way, e.g. eating patterns in the family of a child with anorexia nervosa. It is important to observe family inter-relationships, but the physician may find it hard to preserve his relationship with all members and not take sides.

(5) Psychological Tests

There are various ones available to examine the child's (a) general intellectual functioning; (b) special abilities; (c) educational achievements, e.g. reading, spelling, writing; (d) social maturity.

There are various *projective techniques* which allow the child to express his thoughts and feelings about standardized stimuli; they range from well-organized to less structured (e.g. telling stories about pictures or families, or other human situations). Such tests are task-oriented situations and the child's responses and test behaviour (e.g. motivation, concentration, frustration, tolerance and anxiety) can tell much about his personality and capacity to adapt.

(6) Social Factors

The social and cultural development of the family often dictates what treatment can be offered and limits the necessary treatment. Consider social and economic factors (e.g. stability of employment, housing, family income) and the availability of adequate community facilities (e.g. school, recreation and appropriate social agencies). The family's method of child rearing and their concepts of child behaviour, health and illness must be understood in the framework of their experiences and ethnic and family traditions. Immigrant families are particularly vulnerable in many ways.

THE PHYSICIAN'S ROLE

Accurate diagnosis leads to sound management. General practitioners and paediatricians are confronted with many clinical problems, *most of which represent 'the everyday problem of the everyday child'*. Healthy responses, mild situational reactions and developmental lags, if they are diagnosed and handled wisely encourage the child and family to *grow with confidence*. A sound knowledge of the usual differences in 'normal' behaviour during child development is required to distinguish them from the more serious ones.

Of equal importance is a knowledge of the common psychiatric disorders of adults. The physician should recognize anxiety states, depressive illness, neurotic and personality disorders (particularly obsessive states) in the parents so that he does not confuse them with the special psychological distortions of the parent-child relationship (transactional process). In other words the physician should distinguish between (1) emotional disorder arising in the parent and its impact on the child which may be minimal or maximal, as in a specific identification reaction, and (2) reactive emotional disorders precipitated by the child himself.

The parent who is not able to cope with parenthood will put the child 'at risk'. This should be taken into consideration.

The clinical study of family process will detect the healthy and pathogenic forces operating on the child and prevent 'stereotypic and scapegoating diagnoses' such as 'alcoholic father'; 'inadequate mother'; 'he suffers from an older brother.'

The child psychiatrist therefore works in a medical field, which is highly individual with many complex variables, and which requires considerable flexibility, understanding, tact, tolerance and humility.

All children and parents are attempting to cope as best they can in the circumstances. They are acutely aware of attitudes, the physician's interest in them, and his tolerance. They want doctors whom they can trust and who are reliable and dependable. Children in particular are extremely perceptive and responsive to genuine interest and honesty in their relationships with physicians and can be bewildered when anxiety, fears and conflicts are not perceived, and when treatment is prescribed (e.g. tablets) which seem to have little relation to the problem as they see it.

Regardless of the type of treatment used, the physician must create a relationship which is accepting, empathic, non-critical and non-condemning and yet protective, which permits the patient to trust himself to become aware of the nature of his difficulties. This in itself can be therapeutic.

To the busy practitioner, work with children and parents is often regarded as taking too much time. It is not time but clinical skill which is the issue. Time is ill spent and there are frustrating and unnecessary stresses when treatments are based on inaccurate diagnosis, and become stereotypes which perpetuate disorders, e.g. dependence on drugs.

Whatever is done should create or restore confidence and trust between child and parents, and prevent *undue* dependence on outside help from physicians, and social agencies.

As Hilde Bruch remarked 'One cannot treat a child if one does not respect the parents. The child needs to gain from treatment the conviction that his parents are fundamentally good people.'

PSYCHOTHERAPY

Psychotherapy has been defined as 'the carrying through of a well defined programme for modifying the emotional life and adjustment of a patient through new life experiences and psychological processes which can influence the patient in the direction of health.' A psychotherapeutic programme can be formulated under three headings:

(1) Goals of Therapy: what to treat and why
(2) Areas of Therapy: who to involve and where
(3) Methods of Therapy: how.

(1) *Goals*

Goals should be planned in the light of a comprehensive diagnosis; they should be practical and realistic. Ideally, therapy is indicated for children with emotional disorders that are sufficiently permanent to impede or distort maturational and developmental processes. Many reality factors in the child, family and social situation set limits on what can be achieved, not the least important being lack of therapeutic personnel and facilities. Some children and families may need extensive treatment by specialized psychotherapists, while in other cases more limited intervention may be all that is needed or possible. The physician can help here by establishing a positive relationship and at times offer guidance and advice to help them gain understanding and control.

Symptomatic treatment may be specifically indicated, or used to break a vicious circle where the symptom itself is producing further emotional reaction or secondary gain, and both child and parents together are motivated towards cure. There are dangers because if the symptom is part of a more extensive disorder, the treatment may become an 'attack' leading to the appearance of other disturbances, while symptoms may recur when treatment stops. Concentration on the symptom may establish it more firmly, and when the child and parents relate the treatment procedure itself may become the new focus of conflict leading to other secondary gains and to the exclusion of relevant psychological factors. The true nature of the conflict may be ignored, and effective communication between patients and physician breaks down. However in cases of developmental deviations and situational reactions children suffering from symptoms appreciate direct help and usually respond without 'complications'.

(2) *Areas*

Psychotherapy may be divided into indirect and direct.

Indirect Psychotherapy

Therapy is directed at the child's environment to relieve stress and supply outlets for healthy growth. Work with parents may consist of *helping them as parents—not patients—*to understand the individual child and cope with his practical management. By helping them understand their emotional feelings and perception of the child, which may be confused by lack of knowledge, anxiety and guilt, they are part of, or the sole therapeutic effort to help the child.

More extensive therapy may be needed for the disturbed patient, and later on parents may seek treatment in their own right.

It is most important to understand the problems as the parents see them and, with a deeper understanding of clinical diagnosis, plan treatment and present it to them in a way which is meaningful to their present level of understanding, with the hope that deeper insights will develop. Techniques may include joint interviews between child and parent, or involvement of the whole family therapeutically. Other adults, e.g. grandparents and teachers may be significant and be included with the parents' permission. Where family life is grossly disrupted, alternative placements for the child may be necessary, e.g. fostering, adoption, institutional care.

The child may be helped through his *school*; take account of his assets and deficits, and his social relationships with teachers and fellow pupils. In society, clubs and various social organizations and community resources can provide models for identification and outlets for healthy expression.

Direct Psychotherapy

Indirect psychotherapy of children was the main form of treatment until recent years. Now fuller understanding of development and the child's emotional life make it possible to treat children of all ages. Child psychotherapy is a special skill of child psychiatrists involving intensive training. The methods of psychotherapy are dictated by the child's needs and vary in depth, and duration. Physicians should be aware of the special features and be able to work directly with children in particular cases. Knowledge of child development is essential because the child's fluctuating development and susceptibility to environmental influences at different ages are important variables.

Therapy with children differs from that of adults in that the child, sometimes unwillingly, is brought by someone in his environment, and motivation must be created by the therapist who will need the support and permission of the parents.

Children tend to see their problems and their solutions in their environment, rather than themselves, and have limited powers of self observation. Undisguised feelings may be readily expressed making for technical difficulties. They may readily re-enact their past experiences in the relationship, and on the other hand many quickly enter new experiences. The child imposes changing roles on the therapist. He may be reacted to as a representation of past experiences, or as a new person who actively encourages activities, offers controls or punishes and restrains.

(3) Methods

These can be classified as suppressive, supportive, relationship and expressive.

Suppressive

This is an authoritative directive approach to restore the status quo by diminishing the symptoms. It may work spuriously in the case of the dependent child, and fail with the resistant child. It is usually confined to emergencies or crisis situations and has little use in paediatric psychotherapy.

Supportive

This utilizes guidance, advice, reassurance, encouragement and suggestion. It is used to help the child under stress who cannot cope without support. The therapist permits dependence and regression and also encourages the child to develop those areas where there are difficulties. Various aspects of remedial teaching and speech therapy, occupational therapy could be included here.

Suppressive and supportive therapy do not aim to modify the personality structure but, by relieving stress and aiding areas of function, permit development to proceed. The careful use of tranquillizers and sedation can help as part of comprehensive treatment.

It is important to avoid perpetuating dependence and supporting pathological trends which need more extensive treatment; advice and reassurance are used when specifically indicated.

Relationship and Expressive

The child writes his own script and experiences his anxieties and conflicts through the relationship. The therapist can help him tolerate and master them leading to more healthy integration. Through the therapist's support of reality-testing the child develops self understanding and healthy techniques for adaptation.

The most intensive use of the relationship which can develop is in psychoanalytic psychotherapy or classical child analysis in which unconscious elements are interpreted systematically within a more meaningful transference relationship.

INDICATIONS FOR PSYCHOTHERAPY

Psychotherapy with children is part of a comprehensive plan of treatment adapted to the child's need, and competent judgement is necessary. These forms of psychotherapy are dependent on reasonable and appropriate behavioural expectations set and maintained by children's parents or caretakers.

In general, healthy response and developmental deviations which produce anxiety and conflicts are handled by supportive therapy; situational reactions require a flexible approach.

Fixed neurotic conditions are ideally treated by more extensive therapy. Psychotherapy with some children with personality disorders, psychosis, mental retardation and brain syndromes can be extremely rewarding. Special techniques are needed to establish a therapeutic relationship, and goals should be carefully defined. For example, the angry distrustful, uncontrollable child will need external controls, and limits set by the therapist perhaps including the use of medication as preparation for treatment.

Psychotherapy may be co-ordinated with other medical, educational and social therapeutic measures including behaviour modification techniques and varying degrees of therapeutic help to parents and family. In child psychiatric services child and parents are usually seen by separate workers, psychiatrists, psychologists, social workers, child therapists. In this technique known as 'divide and conquer' both child and parents work in a confidential relationship with their particular therapists and progress is co-ordinated.

Group therapy for children and parents may be of value either in association with individual therapy or alone, but careful selection is needed. Group work with parents, especially those of handicapped children, is particularly valuable, yet a further approach is used in family therapy, namely to understand and work with the family as a unit rather than individual adjustment of family members.

Many countries have a wide range of child psychiatric services as departments of child psychiatry, psychiatric clinics, day centres and residential facilities.

Terms such as child guidance clinic, clinics for children and parents, child and family psychiatry, indicate the orientation of the unit though in fact the basic therapeutic work is common to all.

Specialized units deal with delinquency, psychotic disorders, mental retardation and other problems in paediatrics.

Child psychiatrists have an increasingly important role as consultants to child health, education and social services.

REFERENCES

Anthony, E. J., *Explorations in Child Psychiatry*. (Plenum Press, 1975).

Anthony, E. J., 'The Behaviour Disorders of Childhood', in *Carmichael's Manual of Psychology*, vol. 2, 3rd ed., (Ed. Paul H. Mussen.) Wiley & Sons (New York, 1970), pp. 692-705.

Anthony, E. J. and Koupernik, C. (eds.), *The Child in His Family. The International Yearbook for Child Psychiatry and Allied Disciplines*, vol. 1, 1979. Krieger Publishing Company (Huntington, New York).

Engel, G. L. *Psychological Development in Health and Disease*. W. B. Saunders (Philadelphia, 1962).

Erikson, Erik, *Identity and the Life Cycle*. International Univ. Press (New York, 1967).

*Freedman, Alfred M. and Kaplan, Harold I., (eds.), *Comprehensive Textbook of Psychiatry*. 2nd edn, Williams & Wilkins (Baltimore, 1975). (Child Psychiatry Section).

*Group for the Advancement of Psychiatry, *Psychopathological Disorders in Childhood: Theoretical Consideration and a Proposed Classification*, Aronson, Jason (New York, 1974).

Harrison, Saul I. and McDermott, John, *Childhood Psychopathology*. International Universities Press, 1972.

Hilliard, L. and Kirman, B. H., *Mental Deficiency*, 2nd ed. Churchill (London, 1965).

* Key references.

Howells, J. G., *Modern Perspectives in International Child Psychiatry*, Oliver & Boyd (Edinburgh, 1970).

Josselyn, I. M., *The Happy Child: A Psychoanalytic Guide to Emotional and Social Growth*. Random House (New York, 1959).

Miller, E. (ed.), *Foundations of Child Psychiatry*. Pergamon (Oxford, 1968).

Prugh, D. G., 'Towards an Understanding of Psychosomatic Concepts in Relation to Illness in Children', in A. J. Solnit & S. A. Provence (eds.), *Modern Perspectives in Child Development*. International Universities Press (New York, 1963).

Stuart, H. D. and Prugh, D. G., *The Healthy Child*. Harvard University Press (Cambridge, Mass., 1960).

PAPERBACK CHILD PSYCHIATRY

Some recent publications are very suitable for students.

Wolff, S., *Children Under Stress*. Penguin (1973).

Connell, H. M., *Essentials of Child Psychiatry*. Blackwell (1979).

Rutter, M., *Helping Troubled Children*. Penguin (1975).

Nucombe, B., *An Outline of Child Psychiatry*. University of New South Wales (Sydney, 1972).

APPENDIX 1

A Guide to History Taking from Psychiatric Patients

The purpose of this guide is to help students obtain a history from patients with psychiatric illnesses.

Under *out-patient* conditions, the student should attempt to complete the examination of the patient (including seeing the relatives) in 1½ hours. It is therefore important to concentrate on those aspects of the history which seem clinically relevant. Relatives should usually be seen after the patient's history has been taken.

For *in-patients* the history-taking examination should be conducted in more detail, but following the same general plan. It is often best to do this in two interviews of about an hour each. In addition, relatives must be seen in every case and a full physical examination of the patient made.

REASON FOR REFERRAL

The general practitioner's (or referring) letter should be read first and the main reason for referral at this time defined.

THE HISTORY

Present Complaints

Define the main symptoms and the course of the illness and degree of interference with work, home life, recreation and physical functions such as sleep and appetite. Is there a history suggesting memory impairment?

Family History

Details of parents and siblings. Has any member of the family suffered from 'nervous or mental troubles'?

Personal History

1. *Childhood:* Birth, development. Social and family circumstances. Illnesses.
2. *School. Friends.* Level attained. Scholastic performance. Attitude to work, teachers, other children, games, interests (hobbies).
3. *Work Adjustment:* Nature of job. Is the work record stable, or have there been numerous changes of occupations? Is the patient happy in his present employment?
4. *Marriage:* (if applicable). Husband's occupation. History of marriage. Number of children. Attitude to sex. Menstruation (if unmarried: attitude to opposite sex—whether courting or not, etc.).

Personality (see chapter 6)

Is patient anxiety prone; obsessional (perfectionistic and over-conscientious); shy and withdrawn or sociable; prone to mood swings? What are his interests? Define alcohol consumption. Does he take drugs?

Does present illness seem to be an exaggeration of personality traits?

Past Medical History

Detail accidents, operations and previous psychiatric illness. In which hospitals was the patient treated and when? What treatment was given?

ON EXAMINATION

Mental State

General Appearance and Behaviour

Brief description of appearance and behaviour at interview and mode of communication. Note signs of anxiety, agitation, retardation.

Talk

Describe *form* of patient's talk and note abnormalities.

Mood

Disturbance of mood (depression, elation, anxiety or anger). *Ask for depressive symptoms*, i.e. loss of interest, tiredness, difficulty in concentrating, irritability, sleep disturbance, etc. Note *constancy* and *severity* of any mood disturbance.

Abnormal Thought Content

Describe preoccupations and severity of main symptoms; seek evidence of paranoid delusions or hallucinations. Are there thoughts of suicide? Ask directly concerning phobic and obsessional symptoms.

Orientation, Memory, Intelligence and Ability to Concentrate

These need to be assessed clinically. If abnormalities are suspected, test orientation and memory by questions in Appendix 3.

Insight and Judgment

How does the patient regard his present state? What treatment does he think he will need; does he think he will get well?

Physical Examination

Students should then write a preliminary psychiatric formulation with suggestions for special investigations (if required), and for treatment.

APPENDIX 2

Life Chart

Date.............................

Patient.. Age...........................

AGE	MEDICAL DATA			SOCIAL DATA	YEAR
	Somatic	Psychiatric	Duration of illness		

Note: Spaces can represent years, months or weeks depending upon time relationships of important events.

APPENDIX 3

A Scheme for Memory Testing

1. GENERAL ORIENTATION

Name of Dr testing..

Date.. Time..

QUESTION *VERBATIM ANSWER*

Where are you now?
What is this place called?
What part of town is it in?
What day is it today?
What month is it?
What is the year?
What time is it?

2. MEMORY FOR RECENT PERSONAL EVENTS

QUESTION *VERBATIM ANSWER*

When were you admitted to
  this hospital?

How did you get here?
  (form of transport and route)

Did anybody accompany you?

Did you see another doctor
  before you came here?

What was his name?

Where did you see him and when?

What is my name?
  (make sure you have introduced
  yourself to the patient once or twice
  during previous interviews).

When did I last see you?

3. MEMORY FOR GENERAL EVENTS

QUESTION   *VERBATIM ANSWER*

What important things have happened
in the world recently?

What is the name of the
President of the U.S.A.?

Who was the President
before him?

When did the last war start
and finish?

Which countries were fighting?

Who were their leaders?

What is the name of the
Prime Minister of Australia?
                of Britain?

Who is on the throne of Britain?

How many children has she?

What are their names?

4. MEMORY FOR PAST PERSONAL EVENTS

QUESTION   *VERBATIM ANSWER*

Where were you born?

What year were you born?

What is the name of the school
you went to?

How old were you when you left
school?

Where was your first employment?

How many jobs have you had?

How many years have you been
in your present job?

What year did you get married?

When was your first child born?

When did your mother die?
                        (if applicable)
and your father?

When were you last in hospital?

5. WARD ORIENTATION

To be administered about one week after the patient has been up and about; take the patient round the ward.

QUESTION	VERBATIM ANSWER
Where do you sleep?	
Show me the nearest lavatory.	
Where is the dining room?	
Where is the bathroom?	
Where is the main entrance?	
Are there any other ways out? Where?	
Where is the television?	
Where is the nurse's office?	
What is the name of the nurse in charge of the ward?	
Who sleeps in the same room with you? (or next door)	
Tell me the names of all the other patients you know.	
Do you know the name of any doctors or nurses?	

APPENDIX 4

A Guide to Drugs in Psychiatry

1. MAJOR TRANQUILLIZERS (see chapter 16)

(For the treatment of schizophrenia, organic brain syndromes and mania)

Name	Trade Name (*Tablet size; mg.*)	Usual Adult Dose Range (*mg./day*)	Important Side Effects
Chlorpromazine	Largactil, (10,25,50,100)	75—1,000	Drowsiness, jaundice, fits, photosensitivity hypotension
Thioridazine	Melleril (10,25,50,100)	75—600	Few at usual dosage; impotence
Perphenazine*	Trilafon (2,4,8,16)	6—64	
Trifluoperazine*	Stelazine (1,2,5,10)	6—60	Extrapyramidal Syndrome (see chapter 16)
Haloperidol*	Serenace (0·5,1·0,5·0) (also available in liquid form)	3—20	
Pimozide	Orap (2)	2—10	,,

Diazepam (Valium) can be used systemically for acute brain syndromes (see note on barbiturates, p. 99).

---

* Always give an anti-parkinsonian compound if dosage is *high* or *prolonged* by mouth (particularly in elderly and adolescent patients).

E.g., Orphenadrine	Disipal	50—300
benztropine	Cogentin	0·5—6
benzhexol	Artane	6—10 in divided dosage

2. TRANQUILLIZERS AVAILABLE AS INJECTIONS

Name	Trade Name	Dose/ml.	Ampoules	Route
Chlorpromazine	Largactil	10 mg.	5 ml.	I.M.
		25 mg.	1 ml.	I.M.
Fluphenazine decanoate	Modecate	25 mg.	1 ml.	I.M.
Haloperidol*	Serenace	5 mg.	1 ml.	I.V.
Diazepam	Valium	5 m.g.	2 ml.	I.V.

* Always give an anti-parkinsonian compound if this drug is given by injection. See examples in note to Table 1.

3. MINOR TRANQUILLIZERS
(For the treatment of anxiety, phobic and obsessional symptoms)

Name	Trade Name (*Tablet* (*size; mg.*)	Usual Adult Dose Range (*mg./day*)	Important Side Effects
Diazepam	Valium (2,5,10)	6—30	Ataxia, drowsiness, dependence
Lorazepam	Ativan (1, 2.5)	2—10	
Oxazepam	Adumbran Serepax (10,15,30)	10—30	

Major tranquillizers may be used for low dosage, e.g. Stelazine 1 mg. t.d.s.

4. HYPNOTICS

Benzodiazepines			
Diazepam	Valium (2,5,10)	5—10	
Nitrazepam	Mogadon (5)	5—10	
Flurazepam	Dalmane (15,30)	15—30	dependence
Lorazepam	Ativan (1, 2.5)	1—2.5	
Temazepam	Euhypnos Normison (10)	10—30	

5. ANTI-DEPRESSANT DRUGS (see chapter 12)

Name	Trade Name (*Tablet size; mg.*)	Usual Adult Dose Range (*mg./day*)	Important Side Effects
IMINODIBENZYL DERIVATIVES			
Imipramine	Tofranil (10,25)	75—300	Sweating, dry mouth, drowsiness, constipation, urinary retention, hypotension, extra-pyramidal syndrome, cardiac irregularities.
Amitriptyline	Laroxyl, Tryptanol, Elavil (10,25)	75—300	
Doxepin	Sinequan Quitaxon (10,25)	75—300	
MONOAMINE OXIDASE INHIBITORS			
†Phenelzine	Nardil (15)	30—90	Jaundice, sleeplessness, impotence, hypotension, hypertension
Tranylcypromine	Parnate (10)	20—50	
Isocarboxazid	Marplan (10)	20—60	Important serious side effects*
New anti-depressants See page 76			Reactions with other drugs and some foods

For patients with depression and anxiety or phobic symptoms (see chapter 12) the following are sometimes prescribed:

†Phenelzine (Nardil) + diazepam (Valium)

Tranylcypromine (Parnate) + trifluoperazine (Stelazine) (Parstellin tablets).

Isocarboxazid (Marplan) + diazepam (Valium).

---

* Patients must be warned of side effects, thus:

Your physician has prescribed an effective modern drug for the treatment of your condition. Be sure to follow his directions carefully. Here are a few things to keep in mind while you are taking this medication.

(1) Don't take any other medicines (including cold remedies) without asking your physician.

(2) Don't eat cheese, broad beans or protein extracts. The ingredients of such (especially aged cheeses) may cause a rapid rise in blood pressure.

(3) Don't drink alcoholic beverages without discussing this with your physician.

(4) If you are to receive a general anaesthetic for surgical or other purposes, advise the physician in charge that you are taking this drug.

(5) Report promptly to your physician any unusual headache or other symptoms.

†Patients should be tested to see if they acetylate this drug slowly or rapidly before using the drug. It has been suggested that only slow acetylators respond to phenelzine.

6. PSYCHOTROPIC DRUGS FOR PATIENTS WHO ARE SUICIDE RISKS

Type of Drug	Typical Daily Dose	Lethal Dose	Recommendations
Diazepam (Valium)	15 mg.	reported	Prescribe no more than 2 weeks supply
Tricyclic anti-depressants	150 mg.	10—30 × daily dose	Prescribe no more than 50 × 25 mg. at one time
M.A.O.I.	Varies with drug	Fatalities occur from overdose and reaction with other substances	Patients warned of interactions Prescribe no more than 2 weeks' supply
Phenothiazines	Varies with drug	Fatalities rare	Prescribe no more than 2 weeks' supply

Barbiturates should not be prescribed for these patients.

APPENDIX 5

PAPERBACK PSYCHIATRY

Psychiatry and psychology are popular subjects for the general reader and many paperbacks are available. The following are recommended; some of them have already been referred to at the end of relevant chapters.

Argyle, M., *Psychology and Social Problems*. Pelican, 1972.

————, *The Psychology of Interpersonal Behaviour*. Pelican, 1968.

Beech, H. R., *Changing Man's Behaviour*. Pelican, 1971.

Berne, E., *Games People Play*. Penguin, 1975.

Bowlby, J., *Child Care and the Growth of Love*. Pelican, 1974.

Brenner, C., *An Elementary Textbook of Psychoanalysis*. Doubleday Anchor, New York, 1974.

Bromley, D. B., *The Psychology of Human Ageing*. Pelican, 1974.

Brown, J. A. C., *Freud and the Post-Freudians*. Pelican, 1974.

Comfort, A., *Sex in Society*. Pelican, 1966.

Comfort, A., *The Joy of Sex*. Rigby Ltd., 1975.

Erikson, E. H., *Childhood and Society*. Pelican, 1975.

Eysenck, H. J., *Uses and Abuses of Psychology*. Pelican, 1971.

————, *Sense and Nonsense in Psychology*. Pelican, 1972.

Fordham, F., *An Introduction to Jung's Psychology*. Pelican, 1974.

Foulkes, S. H. and Anthony, E. J., *Group Psychotherapy*. 2nd ed., Pelican, 1973.

Freud, S., *Two Short Accounts of Psycho-Analysis*. Pelican, 1970.

Goffman, E., *Asylums*. Pelican, 1974.

————, *Stigma*. Pelican, 1970.

Hadfield, J. A., *Childhood and Society*. Pelican, 1974.

Hays, P., *New Horizons in Psychiatry*. Pelican, 1971.

Heimler, E., *Mental Illness and Social Work*. Pelican, 1969.

Hinton, J., *Dying*. Pelican, 1974.

Jones, E., *The Life and Work of Sigmund Freud*. Pelican, 1974.

Jones, M., *Social Psychiatry in Practice*. Pelican, 1968.

Kessel, N. and Walton, H., *Alcoholism*. Pelican, 1974.

Marcuse, F. L., *Hypnosis: fact and fiction*. Pelican, 1974.

Mead, M., *Male and Female*. Pelican, 1974.

Miller, G. A., *Psychology: The science of mental life*. Pelican, 1974.

Nathan, P., *The Nervous System*. Pelican, 1973.

Oswald, I., *Sleep*. Pelican, 1974.

Rotter, J. B., *Clinical Psychology*. Prentice-Hall, New York, 1971.

Rycroft, C. (ed.), *Psychoanalysis Observed*. Pelican, 1973.

Ryle, G., *The Concept of Mind*. Peregrine, 1973.

Schwarz, O., *The Psychology of Sex*. Pelican, 1967.

Stafford-Clark, D., *Psychiatry Today*. 2nd ed., Pelican, 1971.

———, *What Freud Really Said*. Pelican, 1968.

Stengel, E., *Suicide and Attempted Suicide*. Pelican, 1973.

Storr, A., *The Integrity of the Personality*. Pelican, 1974.

———, *Sexual Deviation*. Pelican, 1974.

Thomson, R., *The Pelican History of Psychology*. Pelican, 1968.

Walter, W. G., *The Living Brain*. Pelican, 1968.

West, D. J., *Homosexuality*. Pelican, 1974.

———, *The Young Offender*. Pelican, 1974.

Winnicott, D. W., *The Child, the Family and the Outside World*. Pelican, 1975.

Wollheim, R., *Freud*. Fontana/Collins, 1974.

APPENDIX 6
Michigan Alcoholism Screening Test

Questions	Answers with weighted Scoring
1. Do you feel you are a normal drinker? (If patient denies *any* use of alcohol, check here ....)	Yes_____ No _2_
2. Have you ever awakened the morning after some drinking the night before and found that you could not remember a part of the evening before?	Yes _2_ No_____
3. Does your spouse (or parents) ever worry or complain about your drinking?	Yes _1_ No_____
4. Can you stop drinking without a struggle after one or two drinks?	Yes_____ No _2_
5. Do you ever feel bad about your drinking?	Yes _1_ No_____
6. Do friends or relatives think you are a normal drinker?	Yes_____ No _2_
7. Do you ever try to limit your drinking to certain times of the day or to certain places?	Yes _0_ No_____
8. Are you always able to stop drinking when you want to?	Yes_____ No _2_
9. Have you ever attended a meeting of Alcoholics Anonymous (AA)?	Yes _5_ No_____
10. Have you gotten into fights when drinking?	Yes _1_ No_____
11. Has drinking ever created problems with you and your spouse?	Yes _2_ No_____
12. Has your spouse (or other family member) ever gone to anyone for help about your drinking?	Yes _2_ No_____
13. Have you ever lost friends or girlfriends/ boyfriends because of drinking?	Yes _2_ No_____
14. Have you ever gotten into trouble at work because of drinking?	Yes _2_ No_____
15. Have you ever lost a job because of drinking?	Yes _2_ No_____
16. Have you ever neglected your obligations, your family, or your work for two or more days in a row because you were drinking?	Yes _2_ No_____
17. Do you ever drink before noon?	Yes _1_ No_____
18. Have you ever been told you have liver trouble? Cirrhosis?	Yes _2_ No_____

Questions	Answers with weighted Scoring

19. Have you ever had delirium tremens (DTs), severe shaking, heard voices, or seen things that weren't there after heavy drinking?   Yes__2__ No____

*20. Have you ever gone to anyone for help about your drinking?   Yes__5__ No____

*21. Have you ever been in a hospital because of drinking?   Yes__5__ No____

*22. Have you ever been a patient in a psychiatric hospital or on a psychiatric ward of a general hospital where drinking was part of the problem?   Yes__2__ No____

*23. Have you ever been seen at a psychiatric or mental health clinic, or gone to a doctor, social worker, or clergyman for help with an emotional problem in which drinking had played a part?   Yes__2__ No____

24. Have you ever been arrested, even for a few hours, because of drunk behaviour?   Yes__2__ No____

25. Have you ever been arrested for drunk driving or driving after drinking?   Yes__2__ No____

Scores of more than 7 indicate that the patient could be an alcoholic and further assessment is needed.

* Do not include this hospital episode or any outpatient consultation that led to this hospital episode.

INDEX

aetiology of psychiatric illness, 13
alcoholism, 112
amphetamine addiction, 118
anorexia nervosa, 55
Antabuse, 117
anti-depressants, 74, 215
anxiety features, 26, 47; symptoms, 47; *see also* child psychiatry
attempted suicide, 120

barbiturate addiction, 118
behaviour therapy, 60
bereavement, 88
brain syndromes: acute, 98; chronic, 101; *see also* child psychiatry
bronchial asthma, 92; *see also* child psychiatry

certification, 146
child psychiatry, 166; anxiety, 175; autism, 179; brain syndromes, 183; bronchial asthma, 181; child development, 166; childhood disorders, 172; conversion reactions, 175; cretinism, 187; depressive reactions, 176; developmental deviations, 174; dissociative reactions, 175; Down's syndrome, 188; healthy response, 173; management, 195; mental retardation, 186; obsessive compulsive reactions, 176; personality disorders, 177; phenylketonuria, 187; play, 197; psychoneurotic disorders, 174; psychophysiologic disorders, 180; psychotherapy, 201; psychotic disorders, 178; situational reactions, 173
chronic neurotic patients, 44
classification of psychiatric illness, 15
compensation, 50
consultation psychiatry, 161
coping with physical illness, 162
crisis therapy, 59
custodial care, 5
cyclothymia, 28

dependent personality, 28
depressive illness, 67; *see also* child psychiatry
diagnosis of neurosis, 51
drug dependence, 118
drug treatment: of neurosis, 53; in supportive care, 43
drug trials, 140
dying patients, 87

E.C.T., 74
elderly: psychiatric syndromes in, 106
endogenous depression, 70
epidemiology, 10
epilepsy, 86
extrapyramidal syndrome, 136

Freud, S., 19
functional disorders, 16

general practice, 11, 43
grief, 88
group therapy, 59

heredity and psychiatric illness, 13
history of psychiatry, 3
history taking, 30
homosexuality, 151
hypnosis, 60
hypnotics, 138
hypochondriasis, 25, 67
hysterical personality, 26
hysterical symptoms, 49

imipramine group of drugs, 74

Janet, P., 19

Korsakoff's syndrome, 115

learning theory, 60
leucotomy, 6, 81
liaison psychiatry, 161
lithium, 81

maternal deprivation, 157, *see also* child psychiatry
memory testing, 210
menopause, 146
mental apparatus, 20
mental mechanisms. 20
mental state, 33
migration and psychiatric illness, 157
monoamine oxidase inhibitors, 74, 80
mourning, 88

natural history of neurosis, 50
natural history of psychiatric illness, 17
neurasthenic symptoms, 26
neurosis, 48; in general practice, 43
non-restraint, 5

obsessional neurosis, 48
obsessional personality, 24; *see also* child psychiatry
organic disorders, 98

pain, 85
personality: assessment, 23; disorders, 24; *see also* child psychiatry
phenothiazine drugs, 133
physical and psychiatric illnesses, 83
placebos, 142
pregnancy and psychiatric illness, 145
premenstrual syndrome, 143
psychiatric formulation, 39
psychiatric referral: in depression, 7; in neurosis, 54; in sexual problems, 153
psychoanalysis, 58
psychopathic personality, 27
psychopathology, 19, 48
psychosis, 17
psychosomatic medicine, 92
psychotherapy, 57; *see also* child psychiatry
puerperal illness, 146

reactive depression, 70
reassurance, 40

schizoid personality, 27
schizophrenia, 125
sexual problems, 149
side effects: M.A.O.I., 75; tranquillizers, 135
social psychiatry, 154
sociopathic personality, 27
suicide, 120; *see also* attempted suicide
supportive care, 39

tardive dyskinesia, 136
temporal lobe epilepsy, 86
therapeutic community, 6
tranquillizers, 133, 213
transference, 58
treatment: of acute brain syndrome, 100; of alcoholism, 117; of chronic brain syndrome, 104; of depression, 73; of mania, 138; of menopausal symptoms, 147; of neurosis, 52; of paranoid symptoms, 104; of premenstrual syndrome, 145; of psychosomatic illnesses, 95; of schizophrenia, 131; of sexual problems, 150

Wernicke's encephalopathy, 116